T0135601

Benno Schwartz

The natural history of Parkinson's disease in early stages

Logos Verlag Berlin

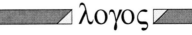

Bibliografische Information der Deutschen Nationalbibliothek

Die Deutsche Nationalbibliothek verzeichnet diese Publikation in der
Deutschen Nationalbibliografie; detaillierte bibliografische Daten sind
im Internet über http://dnb.d-nb.de abrufbar.

ISBN 978-3-8325-2960-4

Logos Verlag Berlin GmbH
Comeniushof, Gubener Str. 47,
10243 Berlin

Tel.:   +49 (0)30 / 42 85 10 90
Fax: +49 (0)30 / 42 85 10 92
http://www.logos-verlag.de

A follow-up on 237 untreated Parkinson patients

Contents

Introduction

The progress made in the therapy of Parkinson's disease since the introduction of the L-Dopa medication has not only influenced the treatment of the illness *per se* but has also, indirectly, stimulated the research concerning its diagnosis and differential diagnosis. Whereas in the nineteen seventies and eighties some authors still regarded hemiparesis, Babinski's sign, sucking and snout reflexes, hyperactive jaw, changes of nucocephalic reflex, impaired vertical gaze or cogwheel visual pursuit as features of idiopathic Parkinson's disease[1,14,15], or confined the main symptoms of Parkinson syndrome (PS) to: resting tremor, bradykinesia and rigidity, nowadays the concept prevails that the cardinal motor symptoms of Parkinson's disease (PD) comprise: bradykinesia, rigidity, tremor and postural instability[2].

Changes took place also in the therapeutical approach of the disease. Still in the eighties and in the beginning of the nineties years of the last century some physicians made the beginning of antiparkinsonian medication depended on the degree of disability caused by PD, and others delayed the beginning of levodopa therapy because of its late complications[3]; nowadays, as a result of the successful therapy of the parkinsonian symptoms, at least in the early stages of the disease, predominates the tendency to begin the antiparkinsonian therapy as soon as possible. This and the looking for a neuroprotective agent had led to the attempt to identify parkinsonian signs and symptoms in the very beginning of the disease and, moreover, to seek signs or markers of the illness in its premotor phase, i.e. before the evident clinical onset.

It is currently commonly accepted that the pathophysiological and biochemical onset of the disease is much earlier than the clinical one[4]. The timespan between the inception of the disease and its clinical outburst has been variously estimated. Whereas some authors suppose that these periods could last as long as 20 to 40 years[5], others, especially based on radionuclide investigations, presume a time lapse of 4 to 6 years[7].

Assuming that the beginning of the medication in the preclinical stage could slow or even stop the development of the disease, there began, especially in the last two decades, the search for biological markers which could lead to identifying the Parkinson's syndrome before its clinical onset.

However, a presymptomatic detection of Parkinson's disease[6], i.e. in the stage of pathophysiological and biochemical changes before the clinical onset, is not yet possible. Certainly, investigations with PET or SPECT that use radioactive substances can make pathological changes in the striatum conspicuous before the clinical symptoms are manifested, as some studies done on the relatives of patients with Parkinson's disease (PD) have shown[7,8], but these methods cannot be used as common screening methods to detect PD in its presymptomatic phase.

Since there are not any biological markers so far which would make it possible to detect the Parkinson's disease in the preclinical stage, it is important to identify the clinical signs and symptoms of Parkinson's syndrome in its very early stages.

James Parkinson stated in 1817[9], that the onset of the disease is slight and nearly imperceptible. Other authors too, such as Calne and Stoessl[10], pointed out that at the onset of the disease the clinical features are frequently mild and vague.

A problem in the identification of the very first signs of PS is the reliability with which they could be assigned to Parkinson's disease. Patients with PD, reporting on the clinical onset of the disease, mentioned various numbers of slight, nonspecific signs and symptoms manifesting along with specific motor parkinsonian symptoms and which, because of that, were considered as of parkinsonian origin. Bulpitt CJ et al.[11] found at least 45 different symptoms attributable to PD. In the past 30 years, some authors interested in the presence of non-motor symptoms in the clinical picture of Parkinson's disease assumed that these symptoms could already be present at the clinical onset of the disease and even appearing before the motor parkinsonian symptoms.

Indeed, the thorough analysis of the medical history of patients with PD could detect signs and symptoms which appeared in some people even before the cardinal motor symptoms became manifested and because of that were regarded as possible forerunners of the disease. All are unspecific signs such as: frozen shoulder, diffuse shoulder or back pain, various paraesthesias without nerval or radicular correlation, mild postural instability, mild changes of the speech, as well as other non-motor symptoms such as smell disturbances, dizziness, constipation, urinary disturbances,

2

internal restlessness, generalized fatigue, diminished spontaneity, some loss of initiative or motivation, mood changes, anxiety, concentration disturbances and mild forgetfulness.

However, some of these symptoms, observed in the months directly before the first manifestation of the PD motor cardinal symptoms, could be considered as forerunners of the disease only when, on the one hand, no other causes for their appearance were found and, on the other hand, there was a continuity between the appearance of these signs and symptoms and that of the motor cardinal symptoms of PD.

Certainly, it would be very interesting to see if patients with one or more such signs also have pathological changes in PET or SPECT investigations with radionuclide substances. This is not yet possible since the patients with those signs usually either do not consult a physician, or the doctor does not take PD into consideration as possible a cause of these signs, or because of economic reasons.

Another problem in the detection of Parkinson's disease in its early stages in elder patients is their age. The prevalence of PD is increasing with age. It is wellknown that approximately 10% of patients are younger than 40 at the clinical onset, whereas in the other 90% the clinical symptoms become manifested after the age of 50[4,12]. As some authors have emphasized[13], the detection of the parkinsonian motor signs in the early stages of PD requires an accurate assessment of the symptoms to differentiate them from the motor symptoms occurring with normal aging.

According to various authors mild extrapyramidal symptoms could be found, too, in normal aging persons[16,17,18,19,20,21,22,23,24].Community-based studies in normal persons older than 65 years showed the presence of mild parkinsonian signs (MPS).These include:bradykinesia, rigidity, mild tremor, or gait disturbance with frequencies between 16.4%[18] and 34.04%[16]. With regard to the age group, according to Bennett DA, Beckett LA et al.,[16] the overall estimated prevalence of MPS in a community population of older people was: 14.9% for the age group 65 to 74 years, 29.5% for the age group 75–84 years, and 52.4% for the age group 85 and older. None of the people with parkinsonian signs found by the aforementioned community-based studies was aware of his parkinsonian signs and symptoms and did not consult a physician for that reason.

The presence of mild extrapyramidal symptoms in otherwise normal elderly persons was explained by the progressive degeneration of the nigrostriatal pathways with loss of neurons and dopamine, which probably would take place in those individuals as a normal aging process[25,26]. It seems that in the very early stages of Parkinson syndrome, in older persons, there exist a mixture of unspecific signs and mild motor symptoms which could be assigned to older age, to other illness, or to the onset of Parkinson syndrome. In fact, in numerous cases these signs are assigned to various illnesses other than to Parkinson's disease and the latter would be taken into consideration only when the motor symptoms became very evident.

The presence of only one parkinsonian motor symptom do not yet allow the diagnosis of Parkinson syndrome. According to London Parkinson Data Bank criteria the Parkinson syndrome is defined by the presence of at least two of the aforementioned cardinal motor parkinsonian symptoms in which one of them is bradykinesia. Certainly, it would be interesting to see in community-based longitudinal studies in subjects with a single parkinsonian motor cardinal symptom if and when more such symptoms would appear, and besides that if in persons with only one parkinsonian motor sign there are in PET or SPECT investigations with radioactive substances already pathological changes in the basal ganglia. In a 57 years old patient with restless legs syndrome and a moderate rigidity treated in own practice no pathological changes by SPECT with[123] I-Ioflupane (DaTSCAN) investigation were found.

Since the paper of Hoehn and Yahr[12], where a thorough analysis of symptoms, progression and mortality on 802 patients with parkinsonism was made, and a now widely accepted clinical disability scale was established, there are few papers which deal with the symptoms and progression of untreated Parkinson's disease[27,28,29,30].

The progress made in the last thirty years in the diagnosis and therapy but also in the clinical evaluation of symptoms of the Parkinson's disease challenges a reevaluation and possibly a new appraisal of clinical signs and symptoms of the disease especially in the early clinical stages.

The aim of this study was to investigate the signs and symptoms of the Parkinson's disease in its early clinical stages and their evolution in untreated Parkinson's disease patients.

Material and Methods

Of the 940 patients with Parkinson's disease examined in the last 15 years, 237 who remained untreated out of various reasons could be followed up. The diagnosis of Parkinson's disease was made on clinical basis. All patients received also a cranial computed tomography or MRI examination of the head. Some patients underwent also a SPECT investigation with ^{123}I-Ioflupane (DaTSCAN) or IBZM.

Once the diagnosis was settled, all the patients unterwent a neurological examination every two or three months in accordance with the UPDRS. This was made each time in on-state. To closer establish the moment of anamnestical manifestation of the first signs and symptoms of PS, the relatives of every patient were also interviewed at the first clinical examination.

The duration of the follow-up varied from 10 weeks up to 86 months in some patients.

Results

All of the 237 patients with untreated PS in this study suffered from idiopathic Parkinson's disease (PD). 87 of them were male and 150 female persons (Fig. 1).

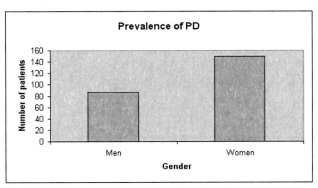

Fig. 1 Prevalence of PD depending on gender

The female/male ratio was 1.72 and therefore different from other studies which noticed a male predominance among the persons affected by Parkinson's disease[31,32]. The cause is not clear. It is simply possible that in this population more women than men became aware of their symptoms and consulted a neurologist.

The age of the patients at the clinical onset ranged from 40 to 93 years, whereas the statistical median age was 70 years. The majority of them (167 or 70.46%) were between 60 and 79 years old at the beginning of the PD with the peak frequency between 70 and 79 years

(Table 1).

Table 1

Age of patients at the clinical onset

Age group	Number of patients	%
40–49	10	4.22
50–59	26	10.97
60–69	77	32.49
70–79	90	37.98
80 and older	34	14.34

The frequency of PD onset in this cohort of untreated patients declined after the age of 80, although it was still higher than in the age group 50 - 59 years.

Compared with the data of Hoehn and Yahr[12] the age-related clinical onset of PD in this study has its frequency peak no more in the age group 50 to 59, but in the age group 70 to 79 years. A higher age-related prevalence of PD was obseved also by other authors[31,16]. The shift to older ages in age-related onset of the disease, already observed by Hoehn & Yahr, seems to become more conspicuous in the recent years. It is possible that in the last years more older persons with PS consult a neurologist because of the progress of therapy in the past 30 to 40 years.

The prevalence of age-related onset was somewhat different in female when compared with male patients. In the age group 40 to 49 years there were 1.5 more men than women, while in the group 80 and older there were more than thrice as many female as male patients (Table 2).

Table 2

Correlation age – gender at the clinical onset

Age group	Men		Women	
	Number	%	Number	%
40–49	6	60	4	40
50–59	9	34.61	17	65.39
60–69	29	37.66	48	62.34
70–79	36	40	54	60
80 and older	7	20.59	27	79.41

It is possible that the greater prevalence of PD in the female patients in the age group older than 80 is related to the higher longevity of women. However the number of patients older than 80 in this study is too small to draw conclusions.

Signs and symptoms of Parkinson Syndrome.

The clinical diagnosis of PS is based on the presence of the motor cardinal symptoms. That is why the main interest of this study was focused on the appearance, frequency and development of these symptoms. As cardinal motor symptoms were considered: bradykinesia, rigidity, tremor, and postural instability.

Anamnestically reported cardinal motor symptoms.

A key point in understanding the pathophysiology of these symptoms is to clarify the way they are appearing in the clinical picture. Usually at the first neurological examination the PD patients are presenting two or more motor cardinal symptoms. It is of interest to see if in the clinical onset of the disease the cardinal motors symptoms are appearing simultaneously or one after the other in a certain sequence.

Certainly, only a long-term observation of persons in whom coincidentally a sole parkinsonian motor symptom was found, would help to identify if additional ones would appear and eventually the sequence of their appearance.

This study attempts to state the appearance and kind of the motor cardinal symptoms in the clinical onset, before the first neurological examination, on the basis of a detailed anamnesis.

Out of the 237 untreated patients with PD 153 or 64.55% considered the appearance of only one motor cardinal symptom as the onset of the disease. The majority of them, namely 118 (77.12%), called tremor as first symptom, 16 claimed bradykinesia, 8 rigidity and 11 postural disturbances. Accordingly, in these patients the tremor was the main reason to consult a physician. The great majority of patients with these symptoms was in the age group 60 to 79 years (Table 3).

Table 3

Cardinal motor symptoms in the anamnesis
Only one symptom

Bradykinesia			Rigidity		
Age group	Male	Female	Age group	Male	Female
40–59	0	1	40–59	0	0
60–79	7	6	60–79	0	6
> 80	0	2	>80	1	1
Tremor			Postural instability		
Age group	Male	Female	Age group	Male	Female
40–59	10	14	40–59	0	1
60–79	33	51	60–79	3	4
> 80	1	9	> 80	2	1

Tremor. Among the patients with tremor as first symptom 38 reported a resting tremor and 80 a postural/action tremor. In this cohort of patients among those who reported anamnestically tremor as first symptom more than twice as many had a postural/action tremor. It is possible that either some of them ignored a rest tremor concurrently present with postural/action tremor or, in fact, a postural/action tremor was the first symptom noticed.

In 35 out of 38 patients with resting tremor this was localized in the hands (20 unilateral and 15 bilateral) and in 3 in the legs. The great majority of the patients with postural/action tremor reported this one localized in the hands (79 out of 80), while 1 had a tremor of of the legs. The postural/action tremor of the hands was observed by 54 patients as beginning bilaterally and by 25 unilaterally (Table 4).

Table 4

Cardinal motor symptoms in the anamnesis

Resting tremor

Age group	Male	Female	Hands		Legs	
			Unilateral	Bilateral	Unilateral	Bilateral
40–59	2	2	3	1	0	0
60–79	13	17	17	11	2	0
>80	0	4	0	3	0	1

Action/postural tremor

Age group	Male	Female	Hands		Legs	
			Unilateral	Bilateral	Unilateral	Bilateral
40–59	8	12	7	13	0	0
60–79	20	34	17	36	0	1
> 80	1	5	1	5	0	0

The female/male ratio of the tremor occurrence was with 1.68 close to the female/male ratio of 1.72 in this study. There was no correlation between the gender and the frequency of the tremor. Nonetheless in patients who reported resting tremor as sole parkinsonian symptom at the clinical onset the female/male ratio reached 1.53,whereas the same ratio was 1.75 in subjects who claimed an action/postural tremor as first manifestation of the disease. It seems that in this cohort of patients the resting tremor was somewhat more frequent in men than in women.

Furthermore, there was no statistical significant correlation between age and and frequency of tremor in every examined age group (regression linear test $p<0.05$) and also no statistical significant difference regarding the frequency of tremor in those groups (one-way ANOVA $p<0.05$). The frequency of the tremor as anamnestically first noticed symptom did not increase concurrently with the age.

Bradykinesia as first cardinal motor symptom was reported by 7 men and 9 women. The great majority of them was in the age group 60–79 years, which was in accordance with the frequency of the age-correlated beginning of the PS in these patients. Out of the 153 patients with anamnestically one motor cardinal symptom at the onset of the disease only 10.45% named bradykinesia. The seldom mentioning of bradykinesia by older patients is possibly also to be a result of the opinion that slower motion is an attribute of older age and not a possible illness symptom. Despite an extensive questioning it was not possible to establish a unilateral beginning of the bradykinesia. All of them reported the bradykinesia as a bilateral symptom. The female/male ratio of patients with bradykinesia as the sole anamnestically motor symptom was 1.28 and so noticeably smaller than the female/male ratio of 1.72 in this study.

Rigidity as first clinical symptom was claimed by 1 man and 7 women and only by patients older than 60 years. A unilateral beginning was denied. The number of the patients who reported rigidity as first symptom is too little to conclude that this symptom was more frequent in female patients.

Postural instability was anamnestically reported as first symptom by 11 patients. Whereas the gender did not influence the frequency, it seems to exist a certain correlation between age and frequency of the postural instability, since 10 out of the 11 patients considering the postural instability as the beginning of the disease were older than 60.

Therefore, in the studied patients the leading sole symptom regarded by them as the beginning of the disease was the tremor. In fact 77.12% of these patients correlated the onset of the disease with the appearance of the tremor and went to see a physician.

Out of the 237 studied patients 84 or 35.45% reported the appearance of more than one cardinal motor symptom as the onset of the disease (Table 5).

Table 5

Cardinal motor symptoms in the anamnesis

Two symptoms

Age group	B+R	B+T	B+P I	R+T	R+P I	T+P I
40–59	2	0	0	2	0	0
60–79	24	6	3	8	0	5
>80	6	2	2	3	0	0

Three symptoms

Age group	B+R+T	B+R+P I	B+T+P I	R+T+P I
40–59	6	0	0	0
60–79	10	1	0	0
>80	1	2	0	0

Four symptoms

Age group	B + R + T + P I
40–59	0
60–79	0
>80	1

Legend
B = Bradykinesia   T = Tremor
R = Rigidity   P I = Postural instability

Three quarters of the patients with more than one cardinal symptom in the anamnesis, namely 63, reported two cardinal symptoms, 20 individuals stated three and 1 four cardinal symptoms. The majority of the patients with two symptoms claimed a combination of bradykinesia and rigidity.

The majority of the patients with more than one cardinal symptom in the anamnesis were in the age group 60–79 years. The gender did not influence the number of cardinal symptoms reported anamnestically.

Anamnestically reported non-motor symptoms

None of the 237 patients with PS in this study claimed spontaneously the appearance of non–motor symptoms like vegetative or sensorial symptoms or named these as reason to consult a physician. The presence of vegetative symptoms was reported only during an intensive personal interview and always accompanying cardinal motor symptoms.

Table 6

Presence of vegetative symptoms in the anamnesis

Age group	Hyper-salivation	Hyper-hidrosis	Miction dysfunction	Constipation	Seborrhoea
40–59	1	0	0	0	0
60–79	6	2	1	1	1
> 80	3	1	1	0	1

Since the hypersalivation is a result of a beginning swallowing dysfunction and not an autonomic nervous system disturbance, it is noticeable that at least in the patients of this study the number of patients which complained on vegetative symptoms was very small (Table 6). In fact, except the patients with hypersalivation, only 8 reported anamnestically vegetative symptoms and just in connection with other motor symptoms. All these patients were older than 60 years. The patients themselves did not make notice on vegetative symptoms and complained about only on questioning. None of the studied patients complained spontaneously about olfactory disturbances.

Cardinal motor symptoms at the first neurological examination

The patients were examinated in accordance to UPDRS in on-state. All patients presented at the first neurological examination with various frequencies 2, 3, or 4 motor cardinal symptoms (Fig.2).

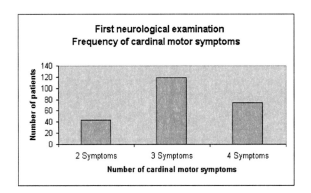

Fig.2 Frequency of the cardinal motor symptoms at the first neurological examination

Actually, out of the 237 patients with PD 41 (17.30%) presented at the first neurological examination 2 main motor symptoms, 122 (51.47%) 3 and 74 (31.23%) 4 cardinal motor symptoms (Table 7).

Table 7

Cardinal motor symptoms at the first neurological examination

Number of symptoms	Number of patients	Kind of symptoms			
		Bradykinesia	Rigidity	Tremor	Posture instability
2 symptoms	41	33	37	12	0
3 symptoms	122	105	119	55	88
4 symptoms	74	74	74	74	74

13

The great majority (82.70%) presented concurrently at the first examination three or four motor cardinal symptoms in the clinical picture.

The bradykinesia was found in 212 patients, jointly with one, two, or three other cardinal motor symptoms. The other 25 had two or three cardinal symptoms but without bradykinesia. The rigidity was obseved in 230 patients along with one, two or three other cardinal symptoms, the postural instability in 162 together with bradykinesia and/or rigidity and/or tremor and tremor in 141 patients as resting tremor and/or action/postural tremor always being accompanied by at least another cardinal motor symptom.

Thus, at the first examination the frequency of the rigidity was a little higher than that of the bradykinesia, and the postural instability was present only concurrently with at least two other cardinal motor symptoms (Table 7).

Since the frequency of PD increased with the age attending its peak in the age group 70–79 years, it was of interest to see if the age could influence the number of main motor symptoms present at the first neurological examination. Correlating the age groups with the number of cardinal motor symptoms (Table 8) the percent of the patients with 2 symptoms reached in patients younger than 60 years 19.44% versus 16.91% in patients older than 60, the percent of those with 3 symptoms 61.11% versus 49.75% and the percent of those with 4 symptoms 19.44% versus 33.33% respectively.

Table 8

First neurological examination

Correlation age – number of cardinal motor symptoms

Age group	Number of patients	Number of patients with:		
		2 symptoms	3 symptoms	4 symptoms
40–49	10	1 (10%)	7 (70%)	2 (20%)
50–59	26	6 (23.07%)	15 (57.69%)	5 (19.23%)
60–69	77	10 (13%)	35 (45.45%)	32 (41.55%)
70–79	90	19 (21.12%)	49 (54.44%)	22 (24.44%)
80 and olde	34	5 (18%)	16 (47.05%)	13 (38.23%)

Although the percentage of patients with three motor symptoms was higher in those under 60, while the frequency of four motor symptoms was higher in those older than

60 years, there was no statistical significant correlations between the age of patients and the number of cardinal motor symptoms at the first neurological clinical examination (regression-linear test $p < 0.05$). There was also no statistical differences at a significant level between the age groups with regard to the number of symptoms at the first neurological examination (one-way ANOVA $p < 0.05$).

To investigate if age and gender could influence the number of main motor symptoms, the age groups and gender were correlated with the number of these symptoms (Table 9).

Table 9

First neurological examination

Correlations age, gender – number of symptoms

Cardinal motor symptoms

Number of patients with	2 symptoms		3 symptoms		4 symptoms	
Age group	Male	Female	Male	Female	Male	Female
40–49	1	0	4	3	1	1
50–59	3	3	6	9	0	5
60–69	5	8	13	20	12	19
70–79	5	13	20	29	10	13
80 and older	1	5	3	12	3	10

The female/male ratio was in patients with 2 cardinal motor symptoms 1.93, in those with 3 symptoms 1.58, and in those with 4 symptoms 1.84. There was no statistical significant differences regarding the number of cardinal motor symptoms between male and female patients in this study (one-way ANOVA $p < 0.05$).

Therefore, that is to assume, that neither the age nor the gender influenced the number of cardinal motor symptoms.

Presence of cardinal motor symptoms at first neurological examination in patients with anamnestically one cardinal symptom at the onset.

To assess the onset of motor cardinal symptoms in the very early stages of PD and to estimate if there is a certain sequence in their appearance, there was analyzed the presence of parkinsonian symptoms at the first neurological examination in the patients which reported anamnestically only one cardinal motor symptom as first manifestation of the disease.

Table 10

Presence of cardinal motor symptoms at the first neurological examination in patients who anamnestically reported only one symptom

Anamnestically one symptom	Number of patients	Timespan clinical onset - first neurological examination								
		Number of motor cardinal symptoms								
		< 1 year			1 to 3 years			4 to 10 years		
		2	3	4	2	3	4	2	3	4
Bradykinesia	16	3	7	4	0	1	0	1	0	0
Rigidity	8	7	1	0	0	0	0	0	0	0
Tremor at rest	38	10	12	10	0	1	2	0	1	2
Action / postural tremor	80	11	20	20	3	7	8	0	7	4
Postural instability	11	2	7	1	0	0	0	0	0	1

None of the patients which reported only one motor cardinal symptom in the anamnesis had also only one motor symptom at the first neurological examination (Table 10).

Of 16 patients which indicated bradykinesia as sole symptom all had bradykinesia together with one, two or three other cardinal motor symptoms. The time lapse between the reported beginning and the first clinical examination was up to 12 months in 14 patients and in two others 2 and 5 years, respectively.

Among the 8 patients which reported only rigidity there was found at the neurological examination in 7 two and in 1 three cardinal motor symptoms. All these patients were examined in less than 12 months from the reported beginning of the illness.

Out of the patients with resting tremor as first anamnestically reported symptom 10 presented at the first clincal examination two cardinal motor symptoms, 14 three,and 14 four motor symptoms. Thirty two of the 38 patients with reported resting tremor unterwent a neurological examination in up to one year, three after 1 up to 3 years and the rest of three up to 10 years after the appearence of the tremor.

In this study 80 patients claimed anamnestically a postural/action tremor as first symptom of the disease. Out of them 14 had at the neurological examination two, 34 three, and the rest of 32 four cardinal motor symptoms. Among these patients 51 consulted a neurologist for the first time in in less than 12 months after the reported appearance of the tremor, 18 after 1 to 3 years and 11 after 4 up to 10 years.

A postural instability as first observed symptom was reported by 11 patients. At the first neurological examination two of them presented 2, seven 3, and two 4 cardinal motor symptoms. All but one consulted a neurologist in less than 12 months and one was examined neurologically after 4 years.

In this cohort of patients, among the cardinal motor symptoms which were anamnestically reported, the rigidity led to a neurological examination in the first year in 100% of patients, followed by postural instability in 91%, bradykinesia in 88%, tremor at rest in 84% and action/postural tremor in 65%. It seems that the tremor was not perceived as a such annoying disability as to consult earlier a neurologist. Hence, 75.15% of the patients who indicated the anamnestically appearance of one motor cardinal symptom as the onset of the parkinsonism consulted a neurologist in up to 12 months. The rest of 24.85% was examined neurologically after 1 up to 10 years.

In patients who anamnestically reported one cardinal motor symptom as the onset of the disease the number of motor cardinal symptoms seemed to increase along with the time elapsed from the onset noticed by patient himself up to the first neurological examination. So, the percentage of the patients with 2 symptoms decreased, whereas that of patients with 3 and 4 symptoms increased, as the first examination took place later (Table 11).

Table 11

First neurological examination

Patients with anamnestically reported one cardinal symptom

Neurological examination	Number of patients	Number of cardinal symptoms		
		2	3	4
up to 1 year	115	33 (29%)	47 (41%)	35 (30%)
1–3 years	20	3 (15%)	8 (40%)	9 (45%)
4–10 years	16	1 (6.25%)	8 (50%)	7 (43.75%)

However, taking into consideration all the 237 patients in this study and correlating the time elapsed from the clinical onset noticed by the patients up to the first neurological examination with the number of cardinal motor symptoms present at the first examination, there was no statistical significant correlation between the disease duration prior to the first examination and the number of main motor symptoms (regression linear test $p < 0.05$).

Hence, is to assume that the patients which considered the appearance of only one cardinal motor symptom as the beginning of the disease ignored the presence of other motor symptoms which were less evident.

Furthermore, it seems there is no definite sequence in the appearance and development of the motor cardinal symptoms. The Parkinson's disease begins not always with the same symptoms, and the appearance sequence of the other cardinal motor symptoms is variable.

Clinical features of cardinal motor symptoms

Bradykinesia. Considered as the most important Parkinson's disease symptom, the bradykinesia could be observed in the very great majority of the patients in this study. To assess the bradykinesia following features of the active movement were considered: initiation time, amplitude, velocity, sequentiality and fluency. Although also other aspects of bradykinesia were delineated, like prolonged time to arrest a false movement, prolonged time to change a motor pattern[33,34], the most characteristic feature is the sloweness of the movement[35]. Because the slowness of motion occurred in parkinsonian patients could begin with a prolonged reaction time to initiate a movement[36], to exclude other causes of a more delayed reaction time and to be sure the task was understood, the patients carried out firstly a motion test.

Since the bradykinesia correlates far better with the delay in the time taken to complete a movement than with the delay in the reaction time[37], and the prolongation of movement time is more substantial and consistent than the slight prolongation of reaction time[38], four aspects of the active movement were taken into consideration in this study to estimate the slowness of motion, namely: amplitude, velocity, sequentiality and fluency. Assuming no impairment of the hand and/or finger joints, the active movement should be repeated 5 seconds always with the same widest amplitude, as rapid as possible, sequential and fluent. The degree of bradykinesia was assessed accordingly to the items 23 to 26 of the UPDRS (subscale III). Whereas amplitude, sequentiality and fluency of the movement are easy to estimate clinically, the estimation of the velocity requires to know the normal values. To ascertain the movement velocity in carrying out finger taps, hand movement, pronation-supination movements of hands and leg agility 341 persons aged between 20 and 94 years without Parkinson syndrome were accordingly examined. None of these individuals had musculoskeletal changes which could interfere with the movement velocity.

According to the age group there was the following distribution:

Age group   20–39 years: 59

                  40–59 years: 100

                  60–79 years: 122

                  > 80 years: 60

The velocity of movement was estimated by the number of the same movement carried out during 5 seconds. In this cohort of individuals the range of movement velocity, independent from age, was:

Finger taps: 11–18/5sec.

Hand movements: 11–18/5sec.

Rapid alternating

movements of

the hands: 11–20/5sec.

Leg agility: 11–17/5sec.

The lowest number of movements carried out in 5 seconds was 11 movements in persons older than 80 as well as in those younger than 40 years. The number of the individuals with a movement velocity of 11/5sec. was the highest in the age group older than 80, while in the individuals younger than 40 years this velocity was seldom noticed. Further, it seemed that the pronation/supination movement was implemented by some persons more rapidly than finger taps or hand movement.

Taking into consideration these data, the cut-off to define the beginning of the bradykinesia with regard to movement velocity was stated at 10 movements/5 seconds. Accordingly, the degree of bradykinesia severity for finger taps, hand movements (hand grips) and rapid alternating movements of hands (pronation/supination movement) was settled as follows:

0 = Normal (11 or more/5sec.)

1 = Mild slowing (10–9/5sec.) with or without amplitude reduction	2 = Moderate slowing (8–7/5sec.) with amplitude reduction
3 = Severe slowing (6–5/5sec.) with evident reduction of amplitude and some disturbances of fluency and sequentiality	4 = Very severe slowing (4 or less/5 sec) with severe amplitude reduction and severe impairment of fluency and sequentiality.

The pronation/supination movements of the hands were estimated firstly during the implementation of the movements with both hands simultaneously (to ascertain if a hand was slower) and afterwards with every hand separately to estimate velocity and amplitude of the movement.

For a semi-quantitative estimation of the movement velocity, it was used a circle-drawing test instead of drawing a spiral. Since the drawing of a spiral, still commonly employed to appreciate the bradykinesia, is dependent not only from the velocity of the movement but also from other factors (personality, academic background, emotional state, etc.), the patients were demanded to draw with a pencil during 1 minute as quickly as possible circles around a disc with a diameter of 12 cm, mobile on a spindle fixed in the middle of a paper sheet. The normal persons achieved 100 to 150 circles in 1 minute but no more than 18 to 20 threads of the spiral. A slowing movement was assumed when the number of circles was under 100.

At the first neurological examination bradykinesia was present in 215 out of the 237 patients in this study. The reduction of movement velocity was not equally represented in the items 23 to 26 of the UPDRS. In 61 patients it was found a slowness in finger taps, as well as in hand movements and rapid alternating movements of the hands. In the other patients there was a slowness only in 2 items either in finger taps and hand movement, or finger taps and rapid alternating movements, or hand movements and rapid alternating movements of the hands. Nevertheless, in patients which could be examined several times, it was found at later examinations a slowness of finger taps, hand movements and rapid alternating hand movements at the same time.The bradykinesia was not alike in upper and lower limbs. Out of 215 patients with bradykinesia at the first neurological examination, only 52 had also an impairment of the leg agility.The others had a slowness of movement only in the upper limbs. No patient had exclusively a slowness of the lower limbs. The bradykinesia was present in some patients only unilateral, in many patients predominantly unilateral, or in a few patients only in one arm. The various localization of the bradykinesia in the early stages of the Parkinson's disease could be the result of a various extention of the pathophysiological changes in the basal ganglia, since the basal ganglia take a non-somatotopic input and produce a somatotopic output[35.]

In this cohort of patients, in the very early stages of Parkinson syndrome the bradykinesia was represented usually by a reduction of movement velocity, which was joined sometime later by an amplitude reduction. None of them presented at the first neurological examination also changes of the finger and/or hand movements fluency or sequentiality The disturbances of fluency and sequentiality appeared only later together with the severe reduction of movement velocity and amplitude. It seems to exist a certain correlation between the severity of bradykinesia and the changes of the movement features.

In the early stages of PD there is not only a slowness of active movements of the limbs but also a poverty of more integrated and complex movements of the limbs and body.

Hypokinesia. Although hypokinesia is regarded as a feature of the more general notion of bradykinesia, the hypokinesia of the arms deserves a special attention, since as a very noticeable objective symptom could be present already in the very early stages of Parkinson syndrome[39].

The hypokinesia of the arms manifests itself as a decreasing of the amplitude or loss of arm swing during walking. The arm swing is a concomitant, automatic, unconscious, movement of the upper extremities during the gait in normal persons. Excluding other causes which could lead to a decreased amplitude up to loss of the arm swing (central or peripherical paresis, orthopedic disabilities, etc.), the unilateral or bilateral hypokinesia of the arm represents an important objective clue in the search of other parkinsonian symptoms.

Out of the 237 patients in this study 205, or 86.5%, presented at the first neurological examination hypokinesia of the arm, unilateral or bilateral (Table 12). In 67 patients the bilateral reduction or loss of arm swing was combined with a general body movement poverty. Generally, the hypokinesia of the arm appears firstly unilateral, becomes later bilateral, and would combine ultimately with a body movement poverty. However, less than 10 patients in this study reported anamnestically a decreased arm swing or a loss of it. The great majority did not noticed a change in the arm swinging.

Table 12

First neurological examination
Presence of the arm hypokinesia

Hypokinesia	Number of patients
No hypokinesia	32
Hypokinesia unilateral	45
Hypokinesia bilateral	93
Hypokinesia of arms with body bradykinesia	67

There was no statistical significant correlation between the gender and the presence, extension and intensity of the arm swing in this cohort of patients (regression linear test $p<0.05$), as well as no statistical significant difference between men and women concerning the frequency of arm hypokinesia (one-way ANOVA $p<0.05$).

Next, there was investigated the correlation between the age and the presence of arm hypokinesia at the first neurological examination.

Bennett DA, Beckett LA et al.[12] found in a community-based study on parkinsonian signs a rising prevalence of reduced arm swing in older age groups not related to the presence of other parkinsonian signs.

Considering the frequency of arm swing reduction or loss in different age groups in the patients of this study, the hypokinesia of the arm was more often seen in older age groups(Table 13).

Table13

First neurological examination
Correlations age – hypokinesia of arm

Age group	Number of Patients	Hypokinesia of the arm			
		0	1	2	3
40–49	10	1 (10%)	1 (10%)	7 (70%)	1 (10%)
50–59	26	5 (19%)	9 (35%)	9 (35%)	3 (11%)
60–69	78	15 (19%)	16 (21%)	25 (32%)	22 (28%)
70–79	89	8 (9%)	18 (20%)	38 (43%)	25 (28%)
80 +	34	3 (9%)	1 (3%)	14 (41%)	16 (47%)

Legend

0 = No hypokinesia

1 = Hypokinesia unilateral

2 = Hypokinesia bilateral

3 = Hypokinesia combined with body bradykinesia

Actually, there was a statistical significant correlation between age and presence of arm hypokinesia (regression linear test $p<0.004$). The prevalence of bilateral arm hypokinesia alone or in combination with body bradykinesia increased with the age. It reached in the age group 50 to 59 years: 46%, in the group 60 to 69 years: 60%, in the group 70 to 79 years: 71%, and in the group 80 and older: 88%. There were statistical significant differences regarding the frequency and intensity of arm hypokinesia between age groups 50 to 59 years versus 70 to 79 years, respectively 50 to 59 years versus 80+ (one-way ANOVA $p<0.05$).

Furthermore, there was considered of interest to look for the correlations between the presence of arm hypokinesia and the other cardinal motor symptoms in the clinical picture of these patients.

Table 14

First neurological examination
Correlations arm hypokinesia – other motor cardinal symptoms

	Number of patients				
	Hypokinesia	Bradykinesia	Rigor	Tremor	Postural instability
No hypokinesia	32	27	30	19	20
Hypokinesia unilateral	45	37	45	27	27
Hypokinesia bilateral	93	84	91	57	63
Hypokinesia + Bodybradykinesia	67	67	67	38	52

Although the reduced arm swing or the loss of it is only an aspect of the bradykinesia, the presence of arm hypokinesia did not always coincide with the bradykinesia estimated according to items 23–26 of the UPDRS. In 32 patients there was no arm swing reduction during the gait, whereas 27 out of them had a bradykinesia (Table 14). Only in the patients with bilateral hypokinesia and body bradykinesia was a 100% coincidence of the two. In the studied patients the unilateral or bilateral hypokinesia of the arm during walking correlated somewhat better with the rigidity than with the bradykinesia according to items 23 to 26 of the UPDRS (Table 14). It could be possible that armswing reduction or loss represents a disturbance of a more complex motor program than bradykinesia.

Rigidity. The intensity of rigidity was estimated by appreciating the resistance to passive movements in the major joints (item 22 of the UPDRS) on relaxed and, if necessary, diverted patient. The rigidity score as expression of the intensity of the rigidity was the sum of scores of the resistance found on passive movement of neck, arm, and leg muscles.

The frequency of rigidity was higher than that of bradykinesia in this study. At the first neurological examination the rigidity was absent in 4 and present in 233 patients.

The localization, extension and intensity of the rigidity was different in many of the examined patients. Whereas in 83 individuals the rigidity was present with the same intensity both in the neck and in the upper and lower limbs, in the other 150 the intensity was either different in the limbs and neck in the same patient, or the rigidity was present only in one or two ipsilateral limbs (in 21 patients). In 2 patients the rigidity affected only the upper limbs, while in none was localized only in the lower limbs. The presence of rigidity was investigated also electromyographically. The muscle activity was recorded with surface electrodes during active maximal contraction of the muscle, after a complete relaxation of the patient and during a passive implemented movement. In all patients with rigidity muscle unit potentials could be recorded during passive contraction of the examined muscle, and in many also during a seeming complete relaxation of this one.

The pathophysiology of rigidity is yet not known. Some studies showed that the passive stretch of human muscles evokes long latencies stretch reflexes which are enhanced in PD[40,41,42] and could be seen already in the early stages of the disease[44]. The long-latency stretch reflex, which is thought to represent a release phenomenon[37], originates in the neuromuscular spindle, do not use probably pathways traversing the basal ganglia themselves, is mediated transcortical and could be influenced by the cortex[45,46,47,48]. The cortex could influence the parkinsonian rigidity through the corticospinal motor projections[49]. Although there is some correlation between the degree of increase in gain of long-latency stretch reflexes and the degree of rigidity in Parkinson patients to which it contributes[37,43], the hyperactivity of the long-latency stretch reflex is not the only mechanism responsible for parkinsonian rigidity, since among others it correlates poor with the rigidity. According to another theory the rigidity is due to a disturbance in the activity of some spinal interneurons as result of abnormal influence transmitted through descending reticulospinal pathways[48,50].
Anyway, the basal ganglia are involved in the pathophysiology of the rigidity.

Taking into consideration the various localization, extension and intensity of rigidity, as observed in this cohort of patients, it is to assume that, on the one hand, a somatotopic distribution of the neurons and pathways is involved in the appearance of rigidity and, on the other hand, the neurons in the same somatotopic region are not equally damaged or physiologically disturbed. This could explain why in the early stages of PD the rigidity in some patients could be clinically found initially in one limb and later in the both ipsilateral extremities. There is not clear yet if the pathways involved in rigidity are the same as those involved in bradykinesia.

However, the starting point of the bradykinesia as well as of the rigidity is probable the same, namely the basal ganglia.

Tremor. At the first neurological examination the tremor was found in 141 (59.43%) out of the 237 studied patients. Tremor at rest could be observed in 36 (25.53%), postural tremor in 63 (44.68%) and a resting combined with a postural tremor of the hands in 42 (29.78%) patients. Usually, the patients with postural tremor had also an action tremor. In patients with resting tremor this one disappeared when the patient stretched his arms or did a movement. The localization of the tremor at rest was variable. Seldom (in 3 patients) it was found unilateral only in the leg, often in one or both hands, and rare of the head and hands (uni- or bilateral) or head and ipsilateral limbs. Only in one patient was observed a tremor at rest of the chin and all limbs at the same time. The postural tremor observed in 63 patients was in all cases localized in the hands either unilateral (24 patients) or bilateral (39 patients). In the remaining 42 patients with combined resting and postural tremor the localization was in the both hands.

The frequency of the tremor was investigated electromyographically in 50 out of the 141 patients with clinical observed tremor. An EMG was recorded simultaneously with surface electrodes on supine or seated patients from the agonist and antagonist muscles of the tremor limb. There were investigated both the tremor at rest and the postural tremor.

Table 15

Electromyographical tremor analysis

Resting/postural tremor	Number of patients
Present	45
Non present	5

In 5 out of the 50 patients electromyogaphycally investigated no tremor could be recorded, although at the clinical examination a resting or postural/action tremor was noticed (Table 15). Out of the 45 patients in whom a tremor was recorded 7 had a tremor at rest and 38 a postural one. The tremor was electromyographically registered as bursts of muscle unit potentials (MUP) present simultaneously in agonist and antagonist muscles appearing either reciprocally alternating or synchronously. In the EMG registration of the tremor the MUP bursts appeared either with the same latency of time both in the agonist and in the antagonist muscles, i.e. synchronously or reciprocally alternating, that is in the antagonist muscles the MUP bursts came with a delayed time latency compared with those in the agonists, so that the MUP bursts onto the antagonist muscle EMG trace fell between two MUP bursts onto the agonist muscle EMG trace.

Table 16

Electromyographical tremor analysis

Kinds of tremor	Number of patients	Reciprocal alternating	Synchronous
Tremor at rest	7	4	3
Postural tremor	38	17	21

There was no great differences between the number of patients with reciprocal alternating and those with sychronously appearing MUP bursts in EMG, and there was also no correlation between the clinical type of tremor and the electromyographical aspects (Table 16). The electromyographical correlation of the tremor at rest as well as of the postural tremor could be with reciprocal alternating but also with synchronous MUP bursts onto EMG traces. Why in some patients the MUP bursts are appearing at the same time in the agonist and in the antagonist muscles, whereas in others the same MUP bursts are appearing in the antagonist muscles with a delayed time latency is not yet known.

The number of bursts/sec. was different in electromyographically investigated patients (Table 17).

Table 17

Electromyographical tremor analysis
Frequency of MUP bursts/sec.

Kind of tremor	MUP bursts/sec.		
		Reciprocal alternating	Synchronous
	Frequency	Number of patients	Number of patients
Tremor at rest	5–6	4	2
	8	1	0
Postural tremor	4–6	11	13
	6–8	5	7
	9	1	1

The number of MUP bursts/sec. in patients with resting tremor electromyographically investigated varied between 5 to 8 with a statistical mean value of 6 (SD=1.15) and a median value of 6. The number of MUP bursts/sec. in individuals with postural tremor electromyographically assessed was in the range 4-9 with a mean value of 6.18 (SD=1.17) and a median value of 5.75. There was no statistical significant differences in the number of MUP bursts/sec. between the tremor at rest and the postural tremor in the electromyographically investigated patients in this study (one-way ANOVA p<0.05). Furthermore, there was no statistical difference on a significant level between the reciprocal alternating and synchronous tremor with respect to the number of MUP bursts/sec. (one- way ANOVA p<0.05). The number of muscle unit potentials per burst (MUP/burst) varied in patients with tremor at rest in a range of 8 to 13 with a mean value of 8.71 (SD=2.13) and a statistical median of 8, while in those with postural tremor the number of MUP/burst was in a range of 3 to 12 with a statistical mean value of 7.18 (SD=1.82) and a median of 7.

Thence, taking into consideration these electromyographycal data, there is to assume that there are no differences between resting and postural tremor in the electromyographically recorded tremor with regard to the number of MUP bursts/sec. as well as to the number of muscle unit potentials recruited per burst.

There are no typical electromyographical features which allows to differentiate between tremor at rest and postural tremor, as other authors too already showed[51].

For long time the description of the symptomatology of Parkinson's disease was dominated by the opinion that the parkinsonian tremor is only a resting tremor. Along with bradykinesia, rigidity and postural instability it was the tremor at rest - and only this form of tremor - which was regarded as cardinal motor symptom of the PD. However in the past 2 to 3 decades various authors emphasized that the tremor in Parkinson's disease could appear as resting, postural and/or kinetic tremor[37,52,53]. Koller et al.[52] found in a group of 50 untreated parkinsonian patients with a complaint of tremor in 92% a postural and in 76% a resting tremor. Among the 141 patients with tremor present at the first neurological examination in this study only one quarter of them had a tremor at rest, whereas in nearly 45% there was found a postural/action one.

On the basis of these data that is to assume that the notion of parkinsonian tremor is defined not only by the kind of tremor but also, and mainly, by the concurrently presence of other parkinsonian main motor symptoms like bradykinesia, rigidity or postural instability. Moreover, the presence of other cardinal motor symptoms allows to differentiate the parkinsonian tremor from the essential tremor since the last one is not accompanied by other neurological abnormalities[54,55,56].

The pathophysiology of the parkinsonian tremor is not yet clear. It seems that the parkinsonian tremor is different from the physiological tremor as well as from essential tremor, and its central generator is probably localized in thalamus[57].

Axial motor symptoms

Posture. The changes in the posture of patients with Parkinson's disease are well known since the monography of James Parkinson (1817) and the subsequently extensive literature on parkinsonism. Two sorts of body stance changes were delineated: the stooped posture and the leaning to one side. The stooped posture is the most observed postural change in patients with PD and could vary from a mild propensity to lean forward up to a severe flexion of the thoracolumbal spine while standing and walking. As Selby[2] pointed out, presenting also a drawing from Gowers 1893, the moderate bent of the trunk and knees is a characteristic posture of patients with PD, which progress concurrently with other disabilities, and in very advanced cases the trunk can be flexed "to almost a right angle at the lumbar level." The severe bent of the thoracolumbal spine was delineated in the recent literature under the term of camptocormia[58,59,60,61,62,63,64].

The posture of the patients with PD in this study was assessed from the side and the frontal face of the patient, and the intensity of the forward leaning of the trunk was appreciated by estimating the distance between the spinal column at the shoulder level and a fancy vertical through the lumbosacral junction. The ventral flexion of the trunk is present while standing and walking, could be very reduced by leaning against a wall, and disappears in recumbent position.

To assess the disturbances of the body's posture was used the following scale:

0 = Normal erect;

1 = Mild: anteflexion of the trunk up to 10 cm. When observed or asked the patient can correct the posture;

2 = Moderate: anteflexion of the trunk up to 15 cm. When asked can correct the posture partially but only for short time;

3 = Salient: anteflexion of trunk more than 15 cm. The patient cannot at all correct willfully his posture and has a tendency to fall forward. It is why some patients have the tendency to speed their pace when walking just to avoid falling down;

4 = Severe: trunk is in anteflexion of more than 15 cm, the limbs are in semiflexion, the patient has sometimes a tendency to stand and walk digitigrade requiring assistance.

The stooped posture of the patient with PD is neither an increase of the physiological dorsal convexity of the thoracal spine nor a kyphosis. The kyphosis remains unchanged in supine position, or by active or passive leaning against a wall. It is also not a curvature of the dorsal spine but rather an anteflexion of the dorsal and lumbar spinal column in the lumbosacral junction.

Hence, it is more appropriate to use the term camptocormia to delineate the forward flexion of the trunk in patients with Parkinson's disease. The camptocormia is etymologically too a forward bent of the thoracolumbal spine irrespective of its intensity and therefore the term cannot be reserved only for the severe bent spine posture.

Camptocormia is an involuntary, from patients themselves usually not or less perceived, forward leaning of the thoracolumbal spine during standing and walking, which disappears by leaning toward a wall or in recumbent position. In the mild to moderate stage camptocormia can be voluntary completely corrected by patients during staying as well as going. In the forward bent of the thoracolumbal spine following muscles are involved: the ventral musculature of the trunk (rectus abdominis, obliquus externus and internus and transversus abdominis), the primary hip flexors (iliopsoas, tensor fasciae latae, pectineus, rectus femoris) and, at least for the first part of the forward leaning movement, the erector spinae and the deep paravertebral musculature.

The other change of the posture, namely the leaning to one side, delineated by Duvoisin and Marsden[65] as scoliotic posture of parkinsonism, which could be seen on old photographs, is nowadays seldom observed. In own Parkinson databank of 940 patients this type of postural change was observed only in 6 patients during the progress of the disease. None of the studied patients presented a scoliotic posture.

Out of the 237 patients in this study 167 (70.46%) had a normal posture at the first neurological examination. The other 70 had a camptocormia. Among the patients with a normal posture were 101 females and 66 males, whereas among those with camptocormia there were 48 women and 22 men (Table 18).

Table 18

First neurological examination

Correlations age – gender – posture

Age group	Number of Patients	Posture			
		Normal		Camptocormia	
		Men	Women	Men	Women
40–59	36	12	18	3	3
60–79	167	51	72	15	29
80 and older	34	3	11	4	16

Whereas the ratio female/male in this cohort of patients was 1.72, the ratio female/male in the patients with normal posture was 1.53 and the same ratio in the patients with camptocormia was 2.18. There was no statistical significant correlation at $p<0.05$ in chi-square test between gender and the abnormal posture, and no statistical significant difference between males and females with regard to camptocormia (one-way ANOVA $p<0.05$).

The gender do not influence the posture of the patients with PD.

Next was examined the role of the age. The age of the patients varied between 40 and 93 years with a mean of 69.13 ± 10.14 and a median of 70. The age of those with normal posture was between 40 and 93 years with a mean of 67.24 ± 9.78 and a median of 69, whereas the age of those with camptocormia had a range between 40 and 91 years with a mean of 73.21 ± 9.76 and a median of 76 years. Thus, the statistical mean and median age of the patients with abnormal posture was higher than those of patients with normal posture.

The prevalence of the abnormal posture was different when correlated with the age. In the age group 40 to 59 years the percentage of the patients with camptocormia was 16.17%, in the group 60 to 79 years increased to 26.34%, and in the age group 80 and older reached 58.83% (Table 19).

Therefore the number of patients with camptocormia at the first neurological examination was increased concurrently with the age at the disease onset. The statistical evaluation of these data indicated a significant correlation between the age and the presence of camptocormia (regression- linear test $p<0.05$).

Since the abnormal posture of the patients with PD differs from the posture of the aging persons without PD (excluding those with diseases of the lumbosacral region), the age alone cannot explain the camptocormia in the patients with Parkinson's disease.

Table 19

Correlations age at disease onset - posture

Age group	Number of patients	Posture			
		Normal	Percent	Camptocormia	Percent
40–59	36	30	83.33%	6	16.17%
60–79	167	123	73.65%	44	26.34%
80 +	34	14	41.17%	20	58.83%

Further, it was of interest to investigate the possible correlations between the extent and intensity of other symptoms of PS represented by the motor score, respectively the total score of the UPDRS and the presence of abnormal posture. The total UPDRS score (T-score) at the first neurological examination was in this study in a range from 3.5 to 57 points, whereas the motor UPDRS score (M-score) had a range from 2.5 to 48 points. Among the 237 studied patients 110 had a T-score < 20 points and a M-score < 18 points. In this group 90 (81.8%) had a normal posture and only 20 (18.2%) a camptocormia. With one exception the abnormal posture was observed only in the patients with at least a T-score of 13 and a M-score of 9 points on the UPDRS.

In another group of 101 patients with a T-score between 20 and 39.5 points and a M-score between 17 and 33.5 points 70 persons (69.3%) had normal posture and 31 (30.7%) camptocormia. In the last group of 26 patients with a T-score from 40 up to 57 points and a M-score from 29 up to 48 points there were 6 (23%) patients with normal and 20 (77%) with abnormal posture.

That is obviously that the frequency of camptocormia in patients with PD rises along with the increase of the T-score and M-score of the UPDRS. There was a statistical significant correlation between T-score respectively M-score and the camptocormia in patients with PD (regression linear test $p<0.05$).

There was also investigated if the presence of camptocormia at the first neurological examination correlates with the degree of disability estimated with the clinical scale of Hoehn & Yahr.

Table 20

First neurological examination
Correlations clinical stages Hoehn & Yahr – state of posture

Stages H&Y	Number of Patients	Posture	
		Normal	Camptocormia
Stage 1	7	7	0
Stage 1.5	7	6	1 (14.28%)
Stage 2	151	110	41 (27.15%)
Stage 2.5	72	44	28 (38.88%)

Out of the 237 patients in this study 223 (94%) had a bilateral symptomatology accordingly to the   Hoehn & Yahr stage 2 and 2.5 (Table 20). Among those 69 (30.94%) presented a camptocormia at the first neurological examination, whereas in the group of 14 patients with unilateral or unilateral + axial symptomatology the camptocormia was found only in 1 (7.14%) individual and only in the stage 1.5 H & Y. There was a significant statistical correlation between the bilateral localization of the parkinsonian symptoms and the presence of camptocormia (regression linear test $p < 0.05$). Taking into consideration these data, it becomes evident that the camptocormia appeared rather on the background of the bilateral + axial localization of the cardinal motor symptoms.

Although a mild camptocormia was somewhat more frequent in patients with Hoehn & Yahr stage 2.5 (29.16%) than in the Hoehn & Yahr stage 2 (22.5%) (Table 21), there was no statistical significant difference between the frequency of the camptocormia and the degree of its severity in the patients in H&Y clinical stage 2.5 when compared with those in the stage 2 (one-way ANOVA $p < 0.05$). It seems that the presence in the stage 2.5 of the postural instability, which makes the main difference to stage 2 on the H&Y scale, do not influence the presence of camptocormia on a statistical significant level.

Table 21

First neurological examination

Correlations clinical stage H & Y – camptocormia

H & Y Clinical stages	Number of patients	Degree of camptocormia			
		0	1	2	3
Stage 1	7	7	0	0	0
Stage 1.5	7	6	1	0	0
Stage 2	151	110	34	7	0
Stage 2.5	72	44	21	5	2

According to the above presented scale to estimate the intensity of camptocormia the great majority of patients with a bent spine at the first neurological examination had a mild form of camptocormia. Actually, 56 (80%) had a mild anteflexion of the trunk up to 10 cm, whereas 12 (17.14%) a moderate and 2 (2.85%) a rather salient one (bent of the thoracolumbal spine of more than 15 cm).

These data pointed out that the bent spine posture could appear already in the early stages of PD and when present it is in the majority of patients of mild intensity.

The pathogenesis of this abnormal posture is yet unclear. While some see in the camptocormia a result of a primary or secondary myopathy of the paravertebral muscles, others consider it as an axial dystonia, an extreme form of rigidity[58,59,60,63], a selective form of PD[64], a heterogeneous disorder with multiple etiologies[62], the possible result of a non-dopaminergic neuronal dysfunction in the basal ganglia[60,61], or a specific neuronal dysfunction in the brainstem[64].

In fact, camptocormia, when considered only as a severe forward bent spine, is rare in patients with PD, especially in the levodopa era, although it seems that levodopa therapy in most cases do not influence the severe forward leaning of the trunk.

However, considering the camptocormia what it is, namely a less or more intense forward bent of the spine in the lumbosacral region, and taking into account the data in this study, there is to assume that this abnormal posture is more frequent in patients with Parkinson's disease and could be present already in its early stages.

There was also of interest to see if the presence of camptocormia was dependent from the duration of the disease. Some authors noticed the presence of camptocormia (as severe bent of the thoracolumbal spine) 4 up to 14 years after the appearance of other parkinsonian symptoms[58,60,61,62].

In this study the presence of mild to moderate leaning forward of the trunk was noticed already earlier. The mean duration between the reported clinical onset and the noticed camptocormia was 2.46 years (SD±1.57).

Table 22

First neurological examination

State of posture

Posture	Number of patients								
	Reported duration of disease								
	<1 y	1 y	2 ys	3 ys	4 ys	5 ys	6 ys	7–9 ys	10–15 ys
Normal	64	42	25	9	6	6	6	4	5
Camptocormi₂	25	22	7	6	6	2	0	1	1

The forward bent of the thoracolumbal spine was noticed in 28.08% of the patients at the first neurological examination done in less than one year after they and/or relatives observed the first signs and symptoms of Parkinson syndrome (Table 22). The frequency of camptocormia did not increase concurrently with the duration of the disease. There was no statistical significant correlation between the duration of the disease and the appearance of camptocormia (regression linear test p<0.05) and also no statistical difference on significant level concerning the disease duration between patients with and those without camptocormia (Mann-Whitney Test p<0.05).

The severity of the camptocormia, too, was in the studied patients not dependent from the duration of the disease (Table 23)

Table 23

First neurological examination

Camptocormia

Number of patients

Intensity	Duration of the disease in years								
	<1	1	2	3	4	5	6	7–9	10–15
Mild	20	16	5	6	5	2	0	1	1
Moderate	4	6	1	0	1	0	0	0	0
Salient	1	0	1	0	0	0	0	0	0

Therefore, taking into consideration the observations done on this cohort of patients, it can be concluded that the forward leaning of the trunk at the lumbosacral level (camptocormia) could be observed, mainly with mild to moderate intensity, already in the early stages of the Parkinson's disease, its appearance is not dependent from the duration of the illness, and its presence is correlated with the older age of the patients at the onset of the disease, with the bilaterality of the symptoms and with the presence and intensity of the motor cardinal symptoms as expressed in the motor score of UPDRS.

To explain the stooped posture of patients with PD some authors[67] advanced the hypothesis that the purpose of the stooped posture is to prevent falls. Jacobs JV et al.[66] rejected this and showed that the stooped posture, although destabilizing, does not account for abnormal postural responses in PD.

Further, there was also suggested, as aforementioned, that the camptocormia could be the result of a muscle disbalance between the dorsal and ventral musculature of the trunk in which the rigidity of ventral muscles is more intense than that of the dorsal ones and that would lead to the bent spine stance.

To examine the role of the trunk muscles rigidity in the appearance of the camptocormia, the EMG changes in the dorsal and ventral trunk musculature were investigated in 30 de novo patients with PD. The EMG was recorded with surface electrodes with a two-channel EMG device from following muscles: erector spinae, obliquus externus abdomini and rectus abdominis in standing as well as in recumbent position. In all these patients causes of bent spine other than Parkinson's disease could be excluded. All but one were not included in this study about the early stages of PD. Out of the 30 patients 13 presented clinically a normal posture and 17 mild or moderate camptocormia, according to aforementioned classification. The age range of the patients was 54 to 89 years with a mean value of 73.16 years (SD±8.34). The mean age of patients with normal stance was 67.85 years (SD±7.85), whereas that of patients with camptocormia was 77.52 years (SD±6.76). The EMG changes were estimated taking into consideration the presence, number and amplitude of recorded MAP (muscle action potentials) during one second.

Accordingly, the intensity of EMG-changes was classified as follows:
1= slight,
2 = moderate,

3 = obvious,

4 = marked.

All patients electromyographically investigated, those with normal posture as well as those with camptocormia, presented no EMG changes in recumbent position.

Out of the 13 patients with clinically normal posture there was recorded from muscle erector spinae unilateral or bilateral in standing position in 4 no EMG activity, in other 4 a slight and in 5 a moderate one. Only in two individuals there was recorded moderate changes also from muscle obliquus abdominis externus. In none of these patients was found in standing position an EMG activity in the muscle rectus abdominis.

Among the 17 patients with camptocormia 11 had clinically a mild and 6 a moderate forward bent spine. In all but one of these individuals the recorded EMG activity was obvious up to marked in the erector spinae muscle and in 8 of them also in the obliquus abdomini externus. In patients with camptocormia no EMG changes were recorded in standing position from the muscle rectus abdominis.

Thus, in the majority of PD patients with normal stance electromyographically investigated it was found slight up to moderate EMG activity in the erector spinae muscle, while in patients with camptocormia the EMG changes were obvious up to marked, and in nearly half of them was involved also the muscle obliquus abdominis externus. The degree of the EMG changes correlated close with the intensity of camptocormia estimated clinically.

These data proved that in patients with PD and camptocormia there is no muscular dysbalance between dorsal and ventral trunk musculature and therefore this could not be the cause of camptocormia. The increase of EMG activity in the dorsal musculature of the trunk seems to be rather the effect of the forward bent spine stance in these individuals.

That is to presume that the forward bent of the trunk in patients with PD has a central origin, and the increased muscular activity in the dorsal trunk musculature recorded by EMG represents actually an effort of the thoracolumbal musculature to prevent a forward shift of the body's center of gravity. A clue for a central cause of the camptocormia was brought recently by a patient with L-Dopa sensitive Parkinson syndrome Hoehn & Yahr stage 3 and hydrocephalus internus who presented a severe camptocormia and was dependent on walker to go. After the operative therapy of the hydrocephalus internus (shunt) the patient is still walker dependent but the camptocormia has completely disappeared.

The camptocormia can cause a forward shift of the body center of gravity. Hence, there was investigated also the correlations between the changes of the stance and those of postural stability.

Out of the 237 patients studied, at the first neurological examination it was found in 55 (23.20%) a normal posture and a normal postural stability, in 51 (21.5%) camptocormia and postural instability, in 19 (8%) camptocormia and normal postural stability, and in 112 (47.3%) normal posture with postural instability (Table 24).

Table 24

First neurological examination

Correlations posture – postural stability

	Number of patients	Duration of disease in years								
		<1	1	2	3	4	5	6	7–9	10–15
Posture and postural stability normal	55	20	8	8	3	2	1	1	1	1
Camptocormia with postural instability	51	17	14	7	6	4	2	0	0	1
Camptocormia with postural stability	19	8	8	0	0	2	0	0	1	0
Posture normal with postural instability	112	44	4	7	6	4	5	5	3	4

Therefore, in the great majority of the patients (78.5%) the appearance of postural instability was not concurrently with the presence of camptocormia. In patients with camptocormia and postural instability there was no statistical significant correlation between the presence of camptocormia and that of postural instability at the first neurological examination (regression linear test $p<0.05$) There was also no correlation between the intensity of camptocormia and that of the postural instability.

Furthermore, it seems, on the basis of these data, that the duration of the disease until the first neurological examination, estimated on the basis of anamnestically reported onset, do not influence the appearance of camptocormia together with postural instability (Table 24). There was, at least in the early stages of PD, no statistical significant correlations between the duration of the disease and the appearance of camptocormia and of postural instability (regression linear test p<0.05).

Thus, it is to assume that the presence of camptocormia does not cause the appearance of postural instability and vice versa. It is also to presume that the pathophysiology of camptocormia is different from that of the postural instability.

Postural instability. Delineated firstly by Charcot[68,69] in the seventies years of the nineteenth century, the impaired postural stability in Parkinson's disease was regarded as a cardinal motor symptom only in the last forty years. As Litvan et al.[70] pointed out, the postural instability in Parkinson's disease is that one not caused by primary visual, vestibular, cerebellar or proprioceptive dysfunction.

The term postural instability defines an impairment of the equilibrium observed earlier or later in patients with Parkinson syndrome and is manifested as a retropulsion or anteropulsion of the body spontaneous or provoked by pull test, respectively push test. However the disturbance of equilibrium, or the propensity to it, can be observed, in more advanced cases, also by turn round during standing or going.

The pathophysiology of the postural imbalance in patients with Parkinson's disease is yet unknown. For decades the postural instability was, and is even now, regarded as a result of impairment or loss of postural reflexes[12,71]. The impairment of the postural reflexes in Parkinson's disease was firstly presumed by Brock and Wechsler[72]. However as the authors admitted, this explanation was speculative, and moreover they reproduced the viewpoint of Magnus which pointed out that "his animal experiments have disclosed no righting reflexes of the kind described by the authors." In the past 40 years various authors incriminated the disturbances or loss of postural reflexes as cause of the postural instability in Parkinson disease[73,74,75]. However it also possible, as some authors already hypothesized[76], that the impairment of postural reflexes in PD is rather the consequence and not the cause of postural instability.

Dysfunctions of various systems were proposed by authors as possible causes of postural instability in parkinsonian syndrome. Martin (cited by Jankovic[71]) considered the postural instability as result of a dysfunction of globus pallidus, whereas Reichert et al.[77] found in patients with PD a vestibular dysfunction which may contribute to the postural instability. Lakke[78] related the postural instability to disabilities of the axial movement which were considered as an apraxic phenomenon[79]. Steiger et al.[80] correlated the postural instability with other disorders of axial movements (turning in bed, arising from chair, gait, whole body bradykinesia, axial rigidity). According to the latter the disorders of axial movement, gait and postural stability were not dependent on the age of patients at onset of the disease, but correlated with its duration. They found that the postural instability, like other disorders, improved after levodopa treatment in nearly all their patients.

As some authors[81] pointed out, the body's equilibrium is the result of the normal function of afferent visual, vestibular, and somatosensory systems and of normal control of muscle tone and peripheral movement. The postural instability is considered as a motor cardinal symptom in Parkinson's disease only when visual, vestibular, and somatosensorial inputs are normal, and beyond it no central or peripheral paresis or cerebellar dysfunction are present. There is to presume that the postural instability appears as result of a disturbance in the associative areas between the normal sensorial and sensitive inputs and the motor output, which ranges from a delayed reaction time up to a loss of adequate motor reaction. Certainly, pathological changes of sensorial (visual, vestibular) or sensitive (proprioceptives) inputs, as well as pathological changes in the functions of efferent motor systems (rigidity, bradykinesia) can facilitate the appearance of postural instability or aggravate it, but do not cause it. As various authors showed, antiparkinsonian therapies could improve the postural instability[80,82,83,84,85,86,87]. However, as others noticed[88,89], the influence of the antiparkinsonian therapies on the postural instability in parkinsonian patients is reduced. The little improvement of the postural instability under antiparkinsonian therapy leads to the presumption that the postural instability is only partially related to dopaminergic lesions[90], and the dysfunction of other non-dopaminergic pathways may contribute to the appearance of postural instability in PD. The postural instability could be related to the disturbance of the postural control of the trunk[91,92,93] and the cortex could be involved in the control of postural responses[94].

In this study the postural stability was assessed mainly in stand, but it was taken into consideration also the postural stability during gait. Guiding by the item 30 of the UPDRS there was used the following scale to estimate the severity of the postural instability:

0 = Normal;

1 = Mild disturbed, in pull test the patient makes a step backwards to maintain his balance;

2 = Moderate disturbed, in pull test the patient needs to do several steps backwards to hold his balance, recovers by oneself;

2.5 = Evident disturbed, in pull test the patient cannot maintain his balance even by doing some steps backwards and must be caught by examiner. In stand and during gait he needs up to 3 strides to turn round.

3 = Marked disturbed, the body equilibrium is unstable. By pulling on shoulders the patient loses immediately his balance, does no steps backwards, would fall if not caught, has an unsteady gait and needs by walking several short steps to turn round or change direction.

4 = Severe disturbed, the patient is unable to stand or to turn round without assistance.

Among the 237 studied patients 74 had a normal body balance and 163 (68.77%) had a postural instability of various degrees at the first neurological examination. As seen above (Table 24), 55 out of the 237 patients (23.20%) had a normal posture concomitantly with a normal body balance, while other 51 patients or 21.51% had at the same time both an abnormal posture and a postural instability. As already aforementioned, in nearly the half of patients in this study there was no concordance between the presence of postural instability and abnormal changes of posture. Therefore it is to assume, at least in these patients, that the postural instability was not caused by abnormal changes of the stance.

To see if the gender could influence the postural instability, the frequency of this one in men was compared with those in women (Table 25).

Table 25

First neurological examination

Correlations gender – postural stability

Gender	Number of pat.	Postural stability		
		Normal	Abnormal	Percent abnormal
Male	87	31	56	64.36%
Female	150	44	106	70.66%

The frequency of postural instability in female patients was somewhat higher than in men.However, at the first neurological examination there was no statistical significant correlation between gender and frequency of postural instability (regression linear test $p<0.05$) and no statistical significant difference in the frequency of postural instability in male compared to that of female patients with PD (one-way ANOVA $p<0.05$).

There was also of interest to investigate if there is a correlation between the age of the patients with PD and the frequency of the postural instability. In the studied patients there was found some increase of the frequency of postural instability in elder patients. So, the percent number of individuals with postural instability at the first neurological examination was in the age group 40 to 59 years 63.88%, in the age group 60 to 79 years 68.86% and in those older than 80 it reached 70.58% (Table 26).

Table 26

First neurological examination

Correlations age – postural stability

Age group	Number	Postural stability		
	of patients	Normal	Abnormal	Postural instability percent
40–59	36	13	23	63.88%
60–79	167	52	115	68.86%
> 80	34	10	24	70.58%

However, the statistical evaluation proved no significant correlation between the age of the patients at the first neurological examination and the postural instability (regression linear test $p<0.05$). There was also no statistical significant differences with regard to the frequency of postural instability between the age groups 40 to 59 years versus 60 to 79 or versus those older than 80, as well as between the age group 60 to 79 years and the age group 80+ (one-way ANOVA $p<0.05$).

Therefore, that is to assume that the age did not influence the frequency of postural instabilitiy in this cohort of patients.

A close correlation was found at the first neurological examination between the total score of UPDRS (T-score) and especially the motor score of the same scale (M-score), on the one hand, and the postural instability, on the other (Tables 27 and 28).

Table 27

First neurological examination

Correlations UPDRS score – postural stability

T - score	No. of patients	Postural stability		
		Normal	Abnormal	Percent abnormal
< 10	12	9	3	25%
10.1–20	96	41	55	57.29%
20.1–30	68	18	50	73.52%
30.1–40	30	5	25	83.33%
40.1–50	22	1	21	95.45%
> 50.1	9	1	8	88.88%

Legend

T – Score = UPDRS total score

Table 28

Correlations UPDRS motor score – postural stability

M – score	No. of patients	Postural stability		
		Normal	Abnormal	Percent abnormal
< 10	26	20	6	23.07%
10.1–20	127	41	86	67.71%
20.1–30	53	13	40	75.47%
30.1–40	26	1	25	96.15%
40.1–50	5	0	5	100%

Legend

M - Score = Motor score (UPDRS subscale 3 score)

The majority of the studied patients (164 or 69.19%) had a UPDRS total score from 10.1 up to 30 points. Out of them 105 patients, or 64.02%, had also a postural instability at the first neurological examination. The frequency of the postural instability increased concurrently with the number of points of the UPDRS T-score. In fact, the percent frequency of postural instability rose from 25% in patients with a

UPDRS T-score under 10 points progressive up to 95.45% in patients with a UPDRS T–score of 40.1 up to 50 points (Table 27).

The correlation was more evident when the motor score was correlated with the frequency of the postural instability in these patients. Out of 177 (74.68%) patients with a UPDRS motor score from 10.1 up to 30 points 128, or 72.31%, had a postural instability. The postural imbalance was almost always present in patients with a M-score of 30 points upwards. The statistical evaluation (regression linear test $p<0.05$) indicated a high statistical significant correlation between T-score and M-score, on the one hand, and the presence of postural instability, on the other hand. There were also statistical significant differences with regard to the frequency of postural instability between the patients with lower UPDRS T-score and M–score and those with higher ones (one-way ANOVA $p<0.05$).

Although the frequency of the postural imbalance increased along with the T-score and M-score, the postural instability seems not to be a consequence of a high T-score or M-score. In this study a postural disequilibrium was observed also in 25% of patients with a T-score lower than 10 points and in 23.07% of patients with M-score lower than 10 points. In the early stages of the PD, in some patients, the course of the postural instability was temporarily rather independent from that of other motor cardinal symptoms like rigidity or bradykinesia. In these patients it could be observed a certain habituation on the pull test despite unchanged severity of the bradykinesia and of the rigidity.

To investigate if the illness duration could influence the appearance of the postural instability in the early stages of PD, the duration of disease estimated from the anamnestically reported onset until the first neurological examination was correlated with the presence of the postural imbalance at the last one.

Table 29

First neurological examination

Correlations postural instability – disease duration up to first examination

Duration of Disease (in years	Total number of patients	Number of patients Degree of postural instability			
		0	1	2	2.5
<1	88	30	26	11	21
1	66	27	14	9	16
2	32	7	12	6	7
3	15	3	5	2	5
4	12	4	5	2	1
5	8	1	3	2	2
6	6	1	0	3	2
>6	10	2	4	2	2

In the early stages of PD the postural instability, estimated by the pull test, was present in a great number of patients already in the first year after the anamnestically reported onset (Table 29). 65% of the patients in this study had a disturbance of the postural stability one year after the reported clinical onset. This percent rose to 78% after two years, to remain almost unchanged in the patients with a longer disease duration until the first neurological examination.(Fig.3).

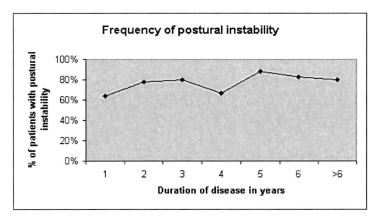

Fig.3 Frequency of postural instability at first neurological examination depending on disease duration.

47

The percentage of patients with an obvious postural instability (the ones which would fall by pull test if not caught) varied between 20 and 33% and did not correlated with the duration of the disease. Although the frequency of postural imbalance was higher in patients with a longer disease duration, there was no statistical significant correlation between the frequency of postural instability and disease duration (regression linear test $p<0.05$), as well as no statistical significant difference in the frequency of postural instability between patients with a disease duration up to 1 year and those with a duration of more than 1 year (one-way ANOVA $p<0.05$).

These data suggest that in the early stages of PD the duration of the disease from the anamnestically noticed clinical onset up to first neurological examination did not influence significantly the appearance of the postural instability.

Further, there was looked for possible correlations between the anatomical localization of the main motor symptoms and the presence of the postural instability. A mild up to moderate postural disbalance could be already observed in some patients with a parkinsonian hemisyndrome, but the frequency was twice, up to three times higher in patients with an additional axial or a bilateral parkinsonian symptomatic. The majority of the patients with PD in this study, i.e. 151 or 63.70%, had a bilateral symptomatic and a retropulsion without falling in the pull test (Table 30).

Table 30

First neurological examination

Correlations anatomical localization of motor symptoms – postural instability

Anatomical localization	No. of patients	Postural stability normal	Postural imbalance	Postural imbalance %
Unilateral	7	5	2	28.5%
Unilateral + axial	7	1	6	86%
Bilateral + moderate postural instab.	165	69	96	58.18%
Bilateral + evident postural instab.	58	0	58	100%

This data suggest that the spread of the parkinsonian symptomatic from unilateral to bilateral could influence the appearance of postural instability in PD.

In 58 patients there was an evident postural instability, according to above described postural imbalance scale. This allows a clear differentiation toward the group of individuals with bilateral symptomatic and moderate postural disbalance (retropulsion with unaided recover in pull test) and let to assume that only in those patients with evident postural imbalance the pathophysiologicaly mechanisms involved are completely present.

Yet, the appearance of postural instability in Parkinson's disease seems to be not conditioned by the presence of reduced dopamine transporter activity in the basal ganglia. Out of a group of 35 patients who were investigated with SPECT and ^{123}I-FP-CIT, 38.46% of those with pathological changes presented no postural imbalance, whereas 46.15% of the patients with normal scan had a postural instability at the first neurological examination.

Since there are evident relations between the anatomical localization of the cardinal motor symptoms and the postural imbalance there was also of interest to check the correlations between the clinical stages according to Hoehn & Yahr and the presence and the severity of the postural instability.

The clinical stages of Hoehn & Yahr are, in fact, based on three pillars:

1. The anatomical localization of the main motor symptoms,

2. The presence and severity of the postural instability,

3. The severity of the cardinal motor symptoms and subsequently the severity of the disabilities in the daily living activity.

In this study the Hoehn & Yahr staging according to UPDRS 1997 with some modifications was applied to estimate the severity and clinical course of the Parkinson's disease.

Accordingly, the following modified Hoehn & Yahr scale was used:

Stage 1 Unilateral localization of at least two of the following cardinal motor symptoms: bradykinesia, rigidity, tremor

Stage 1.5 Unilateral plus axial localization of these symptoms. In some individuals could be found also a mild postural imbalance.

Stage 2 Bilateral localization of at least one or two of the aforementioned motor symptoms with presence of mild to moderate postural imbalance in the majority of individuals (retropulsion without falling in pull test).

Stage 2.5 Bilateral localization of the main motor symptoms with evident postural instability (falling in pull test if not caught by examiner; needs no more than 3 strides to turn around; no spontaneous postural disbalance).

Stage 3 Increased intensity of the bilateral localized cardinal motor symptoms with some more severe impairment of the postural stability (falling in pull test, needs 4 to 6 strides to turn around; first spontaneous signs of postural disequilibrium). The patient is still independent in the activities of daily living.

Stage 4 All cardinal motor symptoms are severe and impending the patient to cope without aid in some activities of the daily living; can stand unassisted, but some need a walking frame to walk.

Stage 5 The parkinsonian symptoms are so severe that the patient need assistance in all activities of daily living. Cannot stand or walk, is wheelchair bound, or bedridden.

The severity of the postural disbalance was correlated with the modified Hoehn & Yahr scale as above presented (Table 31).

Table 31

First neurological examination

Correlations clinical stages Hoehn&Yahr – severity of postural instability

H & Y Stage	Total number of Pat.	Number of patients Degrees of postural instability			
		0	1	2	2.5
1	7	5	2	0	0
1.5	7	1	4	2	0
2	165	69	62	34	0
2.5	58	0	0	0	58

The disturbances of the postural stability increased along with the worsening of the clinical stage Hoehn & Yahr. None of the patients presented a marked or severe postural imbalance according to the above proposed scale to estimate the severity of the postural disbalance. Whereas in the clinical stages 1.5 and 2 the majority of the patients had a mild to moderate postural instability (retropulsion from one to more steps in pull test), in the clinical stage 2.5 all patients had an evident disturbed postural stability, they would fall in pull test if not caught by examiner. So, the appearance of an evident postural imbalance does a clear cut-off between the stage 2 and stage 2.5 on the H & Y scale, and allows also a better estimation of the disease course.

Next, there was of interest to investigate the role of the postural imbalance in the appearance and frequency of falling in early stages of PD.

As numerous authors already showed, falling is a common symptom in Parkinson's disease[95,96,97,98,99,100]. Its frequency reached, according to some authors[95,96] 55-59% and could be influenced by severity and duration of the parkinsonian symptomatic, presence of freezing, dyskinesias, postural and gait disturbances but also by fear of falling.

Of the 237 studied patients 216 (91.13%) reported anamnestically no falling in the time elapsed from the noticed clinical onset up to the first neurological examination. The other 21 (8.87%) accused one or two falls in absence of stumbling or slipping but as a result of the loss of postural balance. All of these 21 patients presented a postural instability at the first neurological examination.

Table 32

First neurological examination

Correlation postural instability – falling

Falling frequency Degree	Number of patients	Number of patients Degree of postural instability			
		0	1	2	2.5
0	216	74	68	30	44
1	16	1	1	6	8
2	5	0	0	1	4

Legend

Frequency of falling 0 = No fall

1 = Less than one fall every 3 months

2 = One fall every 3 months

3 = One fall every month

4 = One fall or more every week

Statistically, there was a high significant correlation between the frequency of falling and that of the postural imbalance (regression linear test p<0.05). Of the 237 studied patients 216, or 91.13%, denied, at the first neurological examination, the occurrence of falling, although 65.74% of them presented, according to aforementioned classification of the postural imbalance severity, a mild up to evident disturbance of equilibrium (Table 32). Only 12 of the 56 patients with evident postural disbalance (in pull test must be caught by examiner to avoid falling) reported anamnestically one or two falls, while 78.57% had no falling. Since only few of them could be followed up more than 48 months, it could not be excluded that at least some developed later PSP.

There was also investigated the influence of the age, and of the gender on the falling in the studied patients. The frequency of falling was correlated to the age and gender as well as to the presence of the postural instability in the persons with falling(Table 33).

Table 33

First neurological examination

Correlations falling – age & gender & postural instability

			Patients with falling					
Age group	Number of patients	Number of pat. with falling	Gender		Degrees of post. instabilit			
			M	F	0	1	2	2.5
40–59	36	1	0	1	0	0	0	1
60–79	167	14	5	9	0	2	3	9
> 80	34	6	2	4	0	1	3	2

In the early stages of PD the percent frequency of the patients with falling reached in the age group 40 to 59 years 2.77 %, in the group 60 to 79 years 8.38%, and the group of patients older than 80   17.64% as reported at the first neurological examination..

Although the number of patients with falling was higher in elder subjects, there was found no statistical significant correlation between the age and the frequency of falling in the early stages of PD (regression linear test p<0.05).

Albeit more women than men claimed falls at the first neurological examination there was also no statistical significant differences between the males and females with regard to the frequency of falling (one-way ANOVA $p<0.05$).

Therefore in the early stages of Parkinson's disease neither the age nor the gender, but the frequency and severity of the postural instability had an influence on the appearance and frequency of the falling.

To assess if the duration of the disease could influence the frequency of falling in patients with PD in early stages, the duration of the disease from the clinical onset until the first neurological examination was correlated with the frequency of falling both estimated according to anamnestically reported data by patients and their relatives.

Table 34

First neurological examination
Correlation disease duration until first examination - frequency of falling

Disease duration	Number of patients	Number of patient with falling	Number of patients Degree of fall frequency		
			0	1	2
<1	88	8	0	6	2
1	67	4	0	3	1
2	31	2	0	0	2
3	15	3	0	3	0
4	12	0	0	0	0
5	8	2	0	2	0
6	6	1	0	1	0
7	1	0	0	0	0
8	1	0	0	0	0
9	3	0	0	0	0
10	4	1	0	1	0
15	1	0	0	0	0

Legend

Frequency of fall   0 = No fall

1 = Less than 1 fall every 3 months

2 = 1 fall every 3 months

3 = 1 fall every month

4 = 1 fall or more every week

The frequency of falling did not increased along with the time elapsed from the reported clinical onset up to the first neurological examination (Table 34). There was also no statistical significant correlation between the disease duration and the frequency of falling (regression linear test $p<0.05$).

According to these data in the early stages of Parkinson's disease the disease duration did not influence the appearance and frequency of falling.

The causes of the postural instability in patients with Parkinson's disease are not yet clear.

Summarizing, the data obtained in this study showed that:

a) The postural instability is present already in the early stages of PD.

b) It appears mainly in patients with bilateral & axial parkinsonian symptomatic.

c) The frequency of the postural instability is not influenced by the gender, or by the age of the patient at the clinical onset of PD.

d) It is not dependent, in the early stages, from the disease duration.

e) Its frequency and intensity rises along with the motor score of UPDRS, and also with the increase of disability according to clinical stages Hoehn & Yahr.

f) In the early stages of PD the postural instability has a great influence on the appearence and the frequency of falling in patients with this disease.

Dysarthrophonia. The speech disorders in Parkinson's disease are various and generally concordant with the disease severity. Some authors found among the initial symptoms an incapacity to control the respiration for the speech, breathiness, monopitch, monoloudness, low loudness, as well as reduced maximum phonation time[101,102,103]. The voice disturbances were attributed in the early eighties of the past century to rigidity and bradykinesia in the orofacial system[104,105]. Subsequent studies[106] showed that the rigidity does not sufficiently explain the labial articulatory difficulties in parkinsonism and pointed out to the dysfunction of the larynx in the genesis of the speech disturbances in Parkinson's disease[107,108,109,110,111,112,113,114,115]. In a some more advanced phase articulation disturbances joined the phonation ones, the speech gets slurred, still understandable, reflecting an increasing dysfunction of larynx, pharynx, tongue and lips[101]. A progression of this dysfunction leads finally to a marked impairment of the speech, which gets nearly unintelligible.

The pathophysiology of dysarthrophonia in Parkinson's disease is not yet completely clear. Whereas rigidity and bradykinesia of the orofacial-laryngeal system play an important part in the genesis of these disturbances, there are probably also other central mechanisms involved. Critchley[101] mentioned that experimental and therapeutic lesions of the inferior medial portion of the ventro-lateral thalamus could influence the initiation, respiratory control, rate and prosody of the speech, whereas other reported data are speaking in favor of the existence of a central pattern generator for the speech movement coordination[116,117].

In this study there was investigated the presence, prevalence, and intensity of the dysarthrophonia in the early stages of the PD and in its correlations with the other motor cardinal symptoms of the disease. The estimation of their intensity was made according to the UPDRS item 18.

Whereas Hoehn & Yahr[12] found among the initial symptoms of 183 patients with primary parkinsonism only in 7 speech disturbances, later reports emphasized the high frequency of voice dysfunction in PD[118].

In the patients of this study there were observed especially changes of the phonation. The voice became rougher, hoarse, breathiness, the pitch and loudness had a limited variability, the loudness of the voice got reduced. However not all these changes in the phonation was present simultaneously in the same patient.It is worthy of notice that in this cohort of patients the majority of them, or their relatives, do not spontaneously claimed themselves about disturbances of the speech, but only on enquiry, during the personal interview.

Hence, if not spontaneously reported, the existence of speech changes must be systematically demanded.

The degree of speech disturbances was estimated according to UPDRS subscale 2 item 5 and subscale 3 item 18, respectively. Severe impairment of speech was not observed in the early stages of PD.

Out of the 237 studied patients 102 (43%) reported at the first neurological examination, the presence of speech changes along with other motor symptoms. The rest of 135 patients, or 57%, and their relatives did not noticed speech changes in the first 1-2 years after the clinical onset.

In 42% of the cases there was a concordance concerning the speech disturbances between the assessement of the patients and relatives (speech ADL) and those of the examiner (Table 35).

Table 35

First neurological examination

Correlations speech ADL – speech motor examination

	Number of patients				
	Degrees of speech disturbances				
	0	1	2	3	4
Speech ADL	135	93	9	0	0
Speech at motor examination	108	113	16	0	0

At the first neurological examination a normal voice was found in only 108 (46%) of the patients with PD, whereas 129 (54%) had speech disturbances. In this respect, these data which are referring only to patients in early stages of PD are different from those of other authors[119], who indicated a frequency of more than 70%. Other 36 patients which believed to have a normal voice but actually it was changed, did not remarked the changes until the neurological examination. In 9 patients which reported speech changes at the personal interview there was found no disturbances of the speech at the motor examination. Otherwise in 50% percent of the individuals with speech changes the estimation by examiner of the disturbances intensity coincided with that of patients or relatives and in other 16% was higher than those assessed by investigated persons.

The frequency of voice changes reached 57.5% in men and 52.33% in women with a F/M ratio of 1.58. However there was no statistically significant difference between the frequency of speech disturbances in men when compared with that in women (one-way ANOVA $p < 0.05$).

Table 36

First neurological examination
Correlations speech disorders – age, gender

Age group	Number of patients	Men Degree of speech disturbances				Women Degree of speech disturbances			
		0	1	2	3	0	1	2	3
40–59	36	8	6	1	0	16	5	0	0
60–79	167	28	30	7	0	48	50	4	0
> 80	34	1	6	0	0	7	16	4	0

Among the 129 patients with speech disabilities 113 could be classified according to UPDRS item 18 as having light, 14 moderate and 2 marked speech disorders.

The frequency of voice disorders was higher in the older patients (Table 36). It reached 33.33% in the age group 40 to 59 years, 54.49% in the age group 60 to 79, and 76.47% in the age group older than 80 years. There was a statistically significant correlation between age and frequency of speech disturbances (regression linear test $p < 0.05$).

Whereas some authors[107] found a 100% correlation of the phonatory abnormalities with the symmetry of trunk and limb rigidity, others[103] observed only few significant correlations between motor components of UPDRS and voice parameters.Because of that, there was of interest to investigate the correlations between the dysarthrophonia and the presence and number of the cardinal motor symptoms in the studied patients.

Out of the patients which presented three motor cardinal symptoms at the first neurological examination 62.65% had speech disturbances. The percent of the patients with speech disturbances was in the group with rigidity and bradykinesia 34.5%, in the group tremor & rigidity 57%, and in the group tremor & bradykinesia 33% (Table 37). It gets evidently from these data that the frequency of speech disturbances is highest in patients with 3 cardinal symptoms and lower in those with only 2 cardinal symptoms in the clinical picture. There was a close relationship, on a statistical high significant level, between the motor score and the presence of voice disorders (regression linear test $p < 0.05$). However this relationship concerned not all main motor symptoms.

There was found a significant statistical correlation between the motor cardinal symptoms but postural instability and the presence of speech disorders (regression linear test $p < 0.05$).

Table 37

Dysarthrophonia

Correlations motor speech disorders – motor cardinal symptoms

at first neurological examination

Complex of symptoms	Number of patients	Degrees of speech disorders			
		0	1	2	3
Tremor & Rigidity& Bradykinesi	166	63	81	22	0
Rigidity & Bradykinesia	61	40	15	6	0
Tremor & Rigidity	7	3	2	2	0
Tremor & Bradykinesia	3	2	1	0	0

Some authors[120] found no dependency of speech intelligiblity on disease severity, duration or motor phenotype.

In this study on patients in early stages of PD there was a statistical difference on a high significant level between the motor score in individuals without speech disturbances and those with light speech disturbances, as well as between the last ones and the patients with moderate speech disturbances (one-way ANOVA p<0.05). The frequency and intensity of voice disorders rose along with the increasing severity of the cardinal motor symptoms and so with the seriousness of the disease.

Taking into consideration only the axial rigidity score expressed mainly by the rigidity of the neck muscles there was no statistical significant difference between the patients without speech disturbances and those with light disturbances, but a significant one when compared the axial rigidity score in subjects with light with those with moderate voice disturbances (one-way ANOVA p<0.05).

Furthermore, there was also looked for the correlations between the localisation of the motor cardinal symptoms (unilateral, unilateral & axial, bilateral) and the presence of the voice disturbances, and thus for the correlations between the frequency and intensity of voice disturbances, on the one hand, and the clinical stages according to Hoehn and Yahr scale, on the other hand.

Table 38

First neurological examination

Correlations speech disturbances – Hoehn & Yahr clinical stages

Clinical stages	Number of Patients	Speech disturbances degrees according UPDRS subscale III				
		0	1	2	3	4
Hoehn & Yahr 1	7	5	2	0	0	0
Hoehn & Yahr 1.5	7	4	3	0	0	0
Hoehn & Yahr 2	165	75	70	20	0	0
Hoehn & Yahr 2,5	58	25	23	10	0	0

In the Hoehn & Yahr clinical stages 1 and 1.5 the percent frequency of speech disturbances reached 35.71% whereas in the stages 2 and 2.5 increased to 55.15%. In the stages 1 and 1.5 (unilateral, unilateral & axial symptoms) there were only mild speech motor changes present, whereas in the stages 2 and 2.5 (bilateral symptoms) there were observed also moderate speech disturbances (Table 38).

Statistically, there was no correlation on a significant level between the speech disturbances and the clinical stages Hoehn & Yahr (regression linear test p<0.05).

Thus, there was no statistical significant correlation between the unilateral or unilateral & axial localization of the motor cardinal symptoms and the presence of speech changes, as well as between last ones and the bilateral localization of the motor symptoms (regression linear test p<0.05).

To assess if the presence of speech disturbances is connected with the severity of the cardinal motor symptoms, the presence of voice changes was correlated with the motor score estimated according to UPDRS subscale III. It was taken into consideration the statistical median value of the motor scores in every clinical stage on the Hoehn & Yahr scale (Table 39).

The speech changes were more frequent and more severe in the patients with a higher motor score. Since, as aforementioned, no statistical significant correlation was found between the presence of speech changes and the spreed of the cardinal motor symptoms (unilateral, unilateral & axial or bilateral), that is to presume that the presence and severity of the speech change correlate rather with the severity of the motor cardinal symptoms.

Table 39

First neurological examination

Correlations motor score in H & Y stages – dysarthrophonia

Speech disturbances degrees

Clinical stage	0 Motor score	1 Motor score	2 Motor score
H & Y 1	3.75	15	0
H & Y 1.5	10.25	22.5	0
H & Y 2	15	23	31.5
H & Y 2.5	18.75	21.5	33.5

Legend

Motor score = Statistical median value of the motor score

In fact, there were in every Hoehn & Yahr clinical stage evident differences in motor score between patients with no speech disturbances (degree = 0) and those with mild (degree = 1) or moderate (degree = 2) voice disabilities when the speech became also slurred. These differences are statistically significant (one-way ANOVA p<0.05). These data are in concordance with the observations of other authors[121] who found in the initial stages the loudness of the voice more impaired than the articulation and fluency.

To estimate the influence of the orofacial rigidity and bradykinesia on the voice disturbances, there was investigated the correlation between the speech disturbances and the rigidity and bradykinesia of the orofacial musculature.

Table 40

Correlations speech disturbances – facial expression

degrees according UPDRS subscale III

		Facial expression			
		0	1	2	3
Speech motor degree	Number of patients	Number of patients	Number of patients	Number of patients	Number of patients
0	108	99	9	0	0
1	99	41	41	14	3
2	30	4	6	14	6

The very great majority of the studied patients with no speech disturbances had also a normal facial expression, while along with increased frequency and severity of voice disturbances rose also the number of patients with minimal up to moderate hypomimia (Table 40).

There was a statistical significant correlation between the speech disturbances and facial expression in these patients (regression linear test p<0.05). However not in all patients the speech disturbances appeared concurrently with changes in the facial expression. In 19% of the studied patients the speech disturbances were present at the first neurological examination without concomitant changes in the facial expression. That is possible that the development of the speech disturbances, at least in some patients, has its own dynamics, differing from that one of the rigidity and bradykinesia of the orofacial musculature.

Functional MRI studies as well as PET investigations of the last years brought important contributions to cerebral localization of the speech and to the pathophysiology of dysarthrophonia in Parkinson's disease. According to various researchers the following cerebral regions are involved in the speech production: the inferior part of the primary sensorimotor cortex (M1) bilaterally, the supplementary motor area, the associative auditory cortex, the cerebellar hemispheres, the right-sided thalamus/caudate nucleus[122,123], the left anterior insula, lateral premotor cortex and left basal ganglia[124], the postcentral gyrus[125] and a larynx-specific area in the motor cortex[126]. In parkinsonian dysarthrophonia there takes place an altered recruitment of the main motor cerebral regions (orofacial M1, cerebellum) and an increased involvement of the premotor and prefrontal cortices (dorsolateral prefrontal cortex, supplementary motor area, superior premotor cortex)[123,127].

On the basis of clinical data recorded in this study there is to presume that in the early stages of Parkinson's disease the appearance and development of the parkinsonian dysarthrophonia expresses clinically the pathological activation of some motor cerebral regions, beginning in the central motor representation of the larynx, and spreading subsequently to other areas of the motor as well as of the premotor cortex. This spreading process is variable in time both interindividually and intraindividually, and could explain also the presence or absence of the changes in facial expression in patients with parkinsonian voice disorders.

Thence, the parkinsonian dysarthrophonia could be defined as the disturbances of voice, articulation,and fluency, which could appear separately or be present all at the same time. In the studied cohort of patients the dysarthrophonia appeared firstly as a voice disturbance, later came in articulation and lattermost fluency disturbances. The transition from voice disturbances to voice & articulation disturbances, to voice & articulation & fluency disturbances was in some patients clear, in others more blurred.

The frequency and intensity of parkinsonian dysarthrophonia could be influenced by the age of the patients, number and severity of the cardinal motor symptoms and the concurrent presence of orofacial rigidity and bradykinesia.

Facial expression. The hypomimia, a common symptom of the parkinsonian syndrome, is a involuntary, spontaneous, diminution of face traits changes, with reduced batting of eyelids and some parted lips, commonly incongruous with some emotional situations of the daily living, which could progress up to a mask-like face.

The Parkinson's disease affects selectively the spontaneous facial expression, whereas facial expressivity related to emotional experience remains relatively intact[128,129].

Whereas some authors[130] could observe in rare cases of Parkinson's disease stage 2 of Hoehn & Yahr scale, i.e. in subjects with bilateral motor symptoms, a persistent hemihypomimia, such change was not found in these studied patients with unilateral, unilateral & axial, or bilateral parkinsonian motor symptoms (clinical stages Hoehn and Yahr 1, 1.5, 2 and 2.5).

The presence and intensity of hypomimia in the early stages of PD was assessed according to item 19 of UPDRS.

Hoehn and Yahr[12] noticed among the initial symptoms of 183 cases with primary parkinsonism a facial masking in 3 patients.

Out of 237 patients in this study, at the first neurological examination, in 144 (60.75%) the facial expression was normal and in 93 (39.25%) the hypomimia was present (Fig.4).

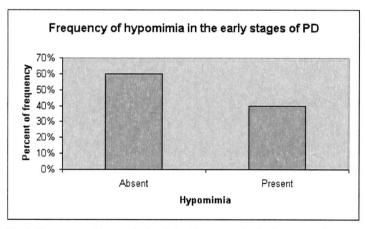

Fig.4 Presence of hypomimia at the first neurological examination

According to these data in the majority of patients with PD in early stages there are no changes in the facial expression (Fig.4).

The frequency of hypomimia increased in the observed patients concurrently with the age (Table 41). Actually, in the age group 40 to 59 years among 36 patients there were 30.55% with hypomimia, in the age group 60 to 79 with 167 patients

36.52% had hypomimia, whereas in the age group older than 80 years with 34 patients the frequency of hypomimia reached 64.70%. There was a statistical significant correlation between age and presence of hypomimia (regression linear test p<0.05).

Table 41

First neurological examination

Correlations age, gender – facial expression

Age group	Number of patients	Men facial expression Degree				Women facial expression Degree			
		0	1	2	3	0	1	2	3
40–59	36	8	3	3	1	17	3	0	1
60–79	167	42	11	8	4	64	18	14	6
> 80	34	3	3	1	0	9	9	6	3

As aforementioned, the ratio female/male (F/M) in this study was 1.72. The ratio F/M concerning the frequency of hypomimia reached 1.76 and therefore close to the ratio F/M ratio in the studied patients. A statistical significant correlation between the frequency of hypomimia and gender was found only in women (regression linear test p<0.05).

To investigate if there are some correlations between the presence of hypomimia and the severity of the motor symptoms, the presence and intensity of facial expression changes were correlated with the motor score at the first neurological examination. The presence and severity of hypomimia went along with the increase of motor score in this study (Table 42).

Table 42

First neurological examination
Correlations hypomimia – motor score

Degree of hypomimia	Motor score
0	16.76 (SD = 7.26)
1	20.74 (SD = 0.79)
2	30.67 (SD = 10.64)
3	31.26 (SD = 14.08)

The presence and severity of hypomimia correlated also statistically on a high significant level with the value of the motor score (regression linear test p<0.05).

To assess the influence of motor symptoms spread from unilateral to bilateral localization, on the presence and intensity of hypomimia it was examined the correlation between the presence and intensity of this symptom and the clinical stages according to Hoehn & Yahr scale.

Table 43

First neurological examination
Correlation clinical stage H & Y - facial expression

Clinical stage	Number of patients	Facial expression degree			
		0	1	2	3
H & Y 1	7	7	0	0	0
H & Y 1.5	7	6	1	0	0
H & Y 2	165	99	34	27	5
H & Y 2.5	58	32	11	11	4

The frequency of hypomimia went concurrently with the spread of motor symptoms from unilateral to bilateral. Whereas the patients with hemiparkinsonismus in this study had no changes of facial expression, and only 1 with unilateral and axial symptoms had also a hypomimia, 40% of the individuals with bilateral symptoms and 44.82% of those with both-side symptoms & postural instability presented a hypomimia at the first neurological examination (Table 43). There was a statistical significant correlation between the frequency of hypomimia and the spread of motor symptoms from one side of the body to the other. (regression linear test p<0.05). It was no statistical significant difference in the frequency of hypomimia between the patients with bilateral motor symptoms (Hoehn&Yahr stage 2) and those with bilateral motor symptoms and postural instability (Hoehn&Yahr stage 2.5) (one-way ANOVA p<0.05).

Summarizing, according to the data of this study, in the early stages of Parkinson's disease the hypomimia is present only in 39.25% of the patients, is more frequent in older individuals, in those with a higher motor score, and with bilateral localization of the motor symptoms. The pathophysiology of hypomimia and its neuropathological correlate is not yet clear. It is speculated that hypomimia correlates neuropathologically with a neuronal loss in substantia nigra, striatum and amygdala; a small loss of neurons in the basolateral nucleus of the latter may contribute to the appearance of this symptom[131].

Arising from chair. The difficulty to arise from chair- a complex coordinated movement involving besides the leg muscles the trunk musculature- is commonly observed in more advanced stages of the Parkinson's disease. In this study there was also looked for the presence of this axial motor symptom already at the first neurological examination.

To estimate the presence respectively the severity of the arising from chair difficulties the follwing scale was used guided by UPDRS item 27:

0 = Normal

1 = Arising independently after one attempt

2 = Arising independently after more attempts

3 = Arise possible only by pushing up with arms from the seat

4 = Unable to arise without help from other person.

Out of the 237 studied patients 163 (68.79%) had at the first neurological examination no difficulties in arising from chair, whereas the other 74 presented such difficulties with various degrees of severity. Of the last ones only 2 individuals need to push up with the arms to arise from seat, 46 could do it after one attempt and 26 after more attempts (Table 44). None of the studied patients need help from other person to arise from chair.

Table 44

First neurological examination
Frequency of arising from chair difficulties

Arising from chair-degrees	Number of patients	% of patients	Men	Women
0	163	68.79%	59	104
1	46	19.40%	14	32
2	26	10.97%	8	19
3	2	0.84%	1	1

Legend

0 = Normal

1 = Arising independently after one attempt

2 = Arising independently after more attempts

3 = Arise possible only by pushing up with arms from the seat

4 = Unable to arise without help from other person

Although difficulties in arising from chair was observed more frequent in female patients there was no statistical significant correlation between gender and those difficulties (regression liniar test $p < 0.05$).

Next, there was investigated the correlation between age and arising from chair. The age did not influence the difficulties in arising from chair in the early stages of the Parkinson's disease. The percent of patients with difficulties in arising from chair was in the age group 40-59ys. 38.89%, it reached 31.74% in the age group 60-79 ys. and in the group older than 80 20.59% (Table 45).

Table 45

First neurological examination
Correlation age – arising from chair

Age group	Arising from chair difficulties degrees				
	0	1	2	3	4
40-59	22	10	4	0	0
60-79	114	31	20	2	0
>80	27	5	2	0	0

Legend
0 = Normal

1 = Arising independently after one attempt

2 = Arising independently after more attempts

3 = Arise possible only by pushing up with arms from the seat

4 = Unable to arise without help from other person.

There were no statistical significant correlation between arising from chair difficulties and the age of patients at the first neurological examination (regression liniar test $p<0.05$), as well as no statistical significant differences regarding the frequency of arising from chair difficulties between the age group 40-59 ys. and that older than 80 (one-way ANOVA $p<0.05$).

Therefore neither the gender nor the age of patients had an influence on the arising from chair in the early stages of the Parkinson's disease.

In this study difficulties in arising from chair were not observed in patients with unilateral or unilateral&axial parkinsonian symptoms but only in those with bilateral symptomatic. However not all patients with bilateral symptoms had also difficulties to arise from chair. In fact 66.21% of them could arise normal. Among them 72.56% were in Hoehn&Yahr stage 2 and 48.27% in stage 2.5. The frequency of the difficulties in arising from chair as well as their severity were higher in patients in the stage 2.5 of the Hoehn&Yahr scale than those in the stage 2. It seems that in the early stages of the PD not only the bilaterality of symptoms but also the severity of these ones could influence the appearance of difficulties in arising from chair. Actually, the frequency of arising from chair difficulties increased along with the motor score values when patients in Hoehn&Yahr stage 2.5 were compared with those in stage 2.

The investigation of the correlations between the UPDRS motor score and the presence of arising from chair difficulties proved a close relationship of the two. There was found a high significant statistical correlation of the arising of chair difficulties to the motor score (regression liniar test $p< 0.001$). However not all motor symptoms involved in the UPDRS motor score had an influence on the arising of chair. The analysis of the correlations between the arising of chair difficulties and each motor symptom included in the UPDRS motor score could prove a close correlation only with the bradykinesia and the postural instability. In fact, there was found a high significant statistical correlation between the arising of chair difficulties,on the one hand, and the severity of bradykinesia as well as that of the postural instability,on the other hand (regression liniar test $p<0.001$).

Accordingly, difficulties in arising from chair could be present already in the early stages of the Parkinson's disease, usually with mild or moderate intensity, are not age or gender depended, but rather from bilaterality of symptoms localisation, and especially from the severity of some motor symptoms as bradykinesia and postural imbalance.

Non-motor symptoms

Whereas the motor symptoms of the Parkinson's disease were delineated by James Parkinson in his monograph "An Essay on the Shaking Palsy" (1817) and refined by Charcot in the latter nineteenth century[68], and although reports on mental impairment in Parkinson's disease appeared already at the beginning of the twenty century[132], only in the second half of the same century began a more detailed investigation of the non-motor symptoms of these disease.

The non-motor symptoms, although very important to further clarify the etiology and pathogenesis of this neurodegenerative disease as well as to appreciate the evolution and prognosis of it, are neither pathognomonic nor specific. The presence of the non-motor symptoms alone, without any of the motor cardinal symptoms, do not permit to put the diagnosis of Parkinson's disease. It is well known that non-motor symptoms as depression or olfactory disturbance could be found in the anamnesis of patients with PD. Nonetheless, there is unknown if these symptoms debuted before, concurrent or after the onset of some motor cardinal symptoms which were not yet noticed by patients.

Because of that there is of interest to investigate the presence of the non-motor symptoms in the early stages of the Parkinson's disease, to estimate their intensity and their evolution.

Psychiatric signs and symptoms

Psychiatric disorders are now regarded as common features of the clinical picture of the Parkinson's disease[133,134].

Already mentioned from the beginning of the twenty century, disorders of the mental state were better described since the sixties years[12,132,135,136].

So found Hoehn and Yahr[12] in their cohort of 806 parkinson patients 4% with moderate to severe depression and 14% with mild-to-moderate organic mental syndrome. However they were already treated patients in various clinical stages, and among them were also patients with encephalitic parkinsonism. These authors reported only in 8 out of 183 patients with primary parkinsonism the presence of depression, nervousness or other psychiatric disturbances among the initial symptoms.

In this study there was investigated the presence of clinical already manifest psychiatric disturbances in early stages of untreated Parkinson's disease. Of the 237 untreated patients with PD 72, or 30.37%, presented at the first neurological examination psychiatric signs and symptoms (Table 46).

Table 46

First neurological examination

Frequency of psychiatric signs and symptoms

	Psychiatric signs and symptoms		
	No	Yes	Percent
Number of patients	155	72	30.37%

The majority of the patients with psychiatric disturbances were females (Table 47). The female/male ratio of the patients with PD and psychiatric symptoms reached 2 and was so obviously higher than the general female/male ratio of 1.72 in this study. There was no statistical correlation between the female/male ratio in patients with PD and the female/male ratio in parkinsonian patients with psychiatric symptoms (chi^2 = -1.06).

Table 47

First neurological examination

Frequency of psychiatric symptoms according to gender and age

Gender	Number of patients with psychiatric symptoms	Age range
Male	24	40–84 years
Female	48	42–91 years

The age range of the female patients with psychiatric disturbances went from 42 up to 91 years and was so nearly to that one of the male patients (Table 47). Whereas in the age group 40 to 59ys. the number of female and that of male patients was nearly the same, the frequency of psychiatric symptoms was among women patients more than twice in the age group 60 to 79 ys. up to three times in the age group older than 80 years than in male subjects (Fig. 5).Actually, in the age group 60 to 79 years there were 33 women and 16 men with psychiatric symptoms, and among the patients older than 80 years there were 11 women and 3 men with these symptoms (Fig. 5).

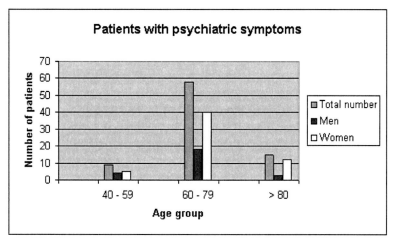

Fig.5 First neurological examination.

Frequency of psychiatric symptoms depending on age and gender

Why in this cohort of PD patients the frequency of psychiatric symptoms was conspicuous higher in women than in men is unclear.

In the studied population of patients the frequency of psychiatric symptoms in various age groups was different from the age correlated prevalence of PD (Table 48).

Table 48

First neurological examination
Correlations age – frequency of psychiatric symptoms

Age group	Age on the clinical onset		Patients with psychiatric symptoms	
	Number of patients	Percent of all patients	Number of patients	Percent of the age group
40–59	36	15.19%	7	19.44%
60–79	167	70.46%	50	29.94%
> 80	34	14.35%	15	44.17%

Although the number of patients with clinical onset at the age older than 80 years remained nearly the same as in the age group 40 to 59 years, the percentage of patients with psychiatric disturbances was more than the twice. In this study the frequency of the patients with psychiatric symptoms in the early stages of the PD increased with the age at onset of the disease and reached its highest value in patients older than 80 years (Fig.6).

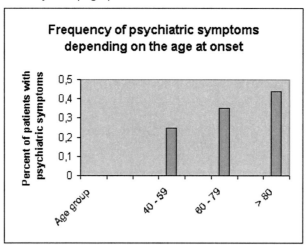

Fig. 6 Frequency of patients with psychiatric symptoms depending on age at onset

Therefore, it is to presume that the age at the onset of the disease plays a certain role in the appearance of psychiatric symptoms in the early stages of Parkinson's disease.

In this study on 237 untreated patients with PD three groups of psychiatric symptoms were observed:

1. Cognitive impairment,
2. Disturbance of mood,
3. Disturbance of behaviour.

Table 49

First neurological examination

Only one group of psychiatric symptoms

Age group	Number of patients	Cognitive impairment		Mood		Behaviour	
		M	F	M	F	M	F
40–59	4	0	1	1	1	1	0
60–79	26	8	12	1	5	0	0
> 80	5	1	3	0	1	0	0

Legend

M = Male

F = Female

The psychiatric investigation done at the first neurological examination identified the three aforementioned groups of psychiatric symptoms, which were present either alone (Table 49) or associated (Table 50). The cognitive impairment alone was noticed in 10.54%, the mood disturbance in 3.79% and behaviour disturbance only in 0.42% of the cases. According to these data the cognitive impairment, when alone present, was the most frequent psychiatric symptom found at the first neurological examination.

However, the majority of the patients with psychiatric symptoms presented already at the first examination a combination of two or three of the abovementioned groups of psychiatric symptoms. In these patients the frequency of the mood disturbance was greater than that of the cognitive impairment (Table 50).

Table 50

First neurological examination
Combined psychiatric symptoms

Age group	Number of patients	Psychiatric disturbances							
		Cognitive& Mood		Cognitive& Behaviour		Mood& Behaviour		Cognitive & Mood& Behaviour	
		M	F	M	F	M	F	M	F
40–59	3	0	0	0	0	1	1	1	0
60–79	24	0	0	0	1	5	5	2	11
> 80	10	0	1	2	4	0	1	0	2

Altogether, in this population of 237 untreated patients with Parkinson's disease at the first neurological examination were found: cognitive impairment in 20.67%, depression in 16.45% and behavior disturbances in 15.61% of the cases (Fig.7).

Cognitive impairment	49
Mood disturbance	39
Behaviour disturbance	37

First neurological examination

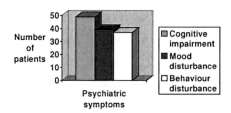

Fig. 7 Psychiatric symptoms at the first neurological examination

1. Cognitive impairment. In the past century numerous authors delineated various aspects of mental status impairment in Parkinson's disease going from light cognitive deficits up to dementia[136,137,138,139,140,141,142]. In the early stages of PD (average disease duration less than 2 years in one study[139]) there were described various deficits in cognitive functions as in the working memory, the verbal and nonverbal memory, the language production, semantic fluency, and in the visuospatial skills both in treated as well as in untreated Parkinson patients. Although already present in the early stages of PD, there was no correlation found between the intensity of cognitive deficits and that of the motor cardinal symptoms[143], and no relationship to the magnitude of rCBF reduction, albeit mean brain hemispheric and regional blood flow were decreased in these patients when compared with normal controls[144]. Numerous others studies are concerned with prevalence, clinical aspects, causes, pathology and pathophysiology of dementia in Parkinson's disease. So, the prevalence of dementia in Parkinson patients varied between 20% and 78% according to authors[132,136,145,146,147,148,149].

Considered in the 1970s by some authors as a subcortical dementia[150] because of similitudes between bradyphrenia and motor bradykinesia, opinion refuted by others[151] - which could demonstrate that the bradyphrenia is not connected to the motor bradykinesia and therefore cannot be attributed to the same basal ganglia disorders which cause the bradykinesia - the dementia in Parkinson's disease is nowadays mainly regarded as a dysexecutive syndrome with impaired attention, disturbances of the executive functions and secondarily impaired memory[147]. Aarsland et al.[152] suggested that the cognitive pattern in Parkinson's disease dementia as well as in the Dementia with Lewy-Body could reflect the superimposition of subcortical deficits upon deficits typically associated with Alzheimer's disease. Whereas earlier dementia in Parkinson's disease was put in connection rather with the presence of the cerebral arteriosclerosis[132,136], nowadays it is regarded more in connection with the age of the patients since dementia is more prevalent in the older Parkinson patients[147].

In the pathophysiology of the dementia in Parkinson's disease was implicated on the neurochemical level, a dysfunction of the dopaminergic, cholinergic, noradrenergic, and serotonergic systems[148,153]. Among these neurotransmitter systems the most disturbed seems to be, according to Emre[147], the cholinergic system.

The pathological background of the Parkinson dementia is not yet clear. Hakim and Mathieson[154] in a postmortem study on Parkinson patients with dementia found, beside a brain weight loss, plaques, neurofibrillary tangles, granulovascular degeneration and cortical cell loss, changes also observed in the Alzheimer disease. Later, clinico-pathological studies in patients with Parkinson's disease and dementia attributed dementia to a subcortical pathology, to an Alzheimer-type pathology, to both of them, to the presence of Lewy bodies in various cortical and subcortical structures, or to factors other than Lewy bodies (review in Emre M, Aarsland D et al. Mov Disorders 2007[149]).

Since neuropsychological investigations proved the presence of cognitive deficits already in early stages of the Parkinson's disease, there was considered of interest in this study to examine to what extent the cognitive disturbances are already present at the routine clinical psychiatric exploration of untreated patients in the early stages of PD, and if and to what extent the deficits are influencing the activity of daily living of these patients.

The presence and intensity of the psychiatric symptoms in patients with early stages of Parkinson's disease, was estimated according to the subscale I of the UPDRS.

The subscale I is rather more focused on the memory disturbance. Starkstein and Merello[155] found that a score of 2 or greater on the UPDRS subscale I had 60% sensitivity and 92% specificity to detect dementia. The sensitivity reached 85% when the MMSE with a score of 23 or lower was included.

In this study the mental state was investigated by a comprehensive clinical psychiatric examination and with the Mini-Mental State Examination[156]. Out of the 72 patients with psychiatric symptoms in this cohort of patients 49, or 68.05%, had mostly mild cognitive impairment manifested as disturbance of the recent memory. This frequency is far off to that reported by other authors[157], who found a frequency of 24% in newly diagnosed PD. The cognitive impairment appeared initially as a frequent, later as a consistent, mild forgetfulness in the activities of daily living and/or in the professional activities. Usually, the presence of this mild forgetfulness was firstly observed by the family, whereas the patient tried to hide or ignore it. Disturbances of the thinking, planning or of the executive functions which influenced the activities of daily living were seldom observed and only with mild intensity in patients with slight cognitive impairment corresponding to score 1 on UPDRS subscale I.

Out of the 49 patients with cognitive deficits at the first neurological examination 25 had only this symptom, while the other 24 presented also a depression and/or a diminished motivation/initiative.

In the studied patients the cognitive deficit as only symptom or associated with mood and/or behavior disturbances was present at the first neurological examination in 35 women and 14 men with PD (Tables 47, 48). The ratio female/male (F/M) was 2.5 and therefore higher as the general ratio F/M of 1.72 in this study. However in the patients with cognitive deficit alone the F/M ratio reached 1.66, while the same ratio attained a value of 3.8 in the patients with cognitive deficit associated with depression and/or motivation/initiative disorders. It seems that among these patients the cognitive impairment was more frequent in females when associated with depression and motivation/initiative loss. However there was no statistically significant correlation between gender and frequency of cognitive impairment (regression linear test $p < 0.05$).

The frequency of patients with PD and cognitive impairment at the first neurological examination increased along with the age. Whereas in the age group 40 to 59 years the percent of cognitive deficits was 5.55%, it attained nearly a four times higher value in the age group 40 to 79 years.

The highest percent number of patients with cognitive impairment occurred in those older than 80 years and reached 38.23% (Table 51).

Table 51

First neurological examination

Age- depending distribution of cognitive deficits

Age group	Number of patients	Number of patients with cognitive deficit	Percent of cognitive deficit
40–59	36	2	5.55%
60–79	167	34	20.35%
> 80	34	13	38.23%

There was a high significant statistical correlation between the frequency of the intellectual impairment and the age at onset in these patients (regression linear test $p < 0.05$). These data confirmed those already known in the literature[147]. When the frequency of cognitive deficit was correlated with the gender and age there was a high significant statistical correlation only in female patients (regression linear test p<0.05).

In 82% of the patients with cognitive impairment the deficit was mild and was estimated with 1 point of the UPDRS subscale I, while in 18% the intellectual impairment was rated with 2 points of the same scale (Table 52).

Whereas the patients with mild cognitive impairment complained a slight forgetfulness with some attention deficit, sometimes noticed by themselves, sometimes by the relatives, which could be usually corrected and did not influenced the activities of the daily living, those with moderate cognitive deficits had a moderate attention deficit, a persistent impairment of the short term memory, evident difficulties in planing and executing, often time desorientation and some problems to cope with the activities of daily living.

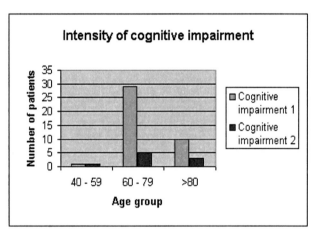

Fig.8 Distribution of cognitive impairment intensity according to age

In this cohort of patients there was found no evident or severe impairment of intellectual functions at the first neurological examination. Although the frequency of mild and moderate cognitive deficits increased along the age (Table 52), there was no statistical significant correlation between age and severity of the intellectual impairment (regression linear test p<0.05).

Table 52

First neurological examination
Intensity of the cognitive deficits

Age group	Number of patients	UPDRS-Subscale I - score			
		1	2	3	4
40–59	2	1	1	0	0
60–79	34	29	5	0	0
> 80	13	10	3	0	0

The great majority of the patients detected with cognitive deficits at the psychiatric exploration underwent also a Mini-Mental State Examination (MMSE).

A MMSE was done in 36 of the 49 patients with cognitive impairment at the first neurological examination. Of them 31 (86%) reached in MMSE a score between 26 and 30 points and in UPDRS subscale I - Intellectual impairment 1 point. Out of the other 5 patients who had on the UPDRS subscale I a score of 2 points one reached a MMSE score of 29, and another 4 patients a score of 25 points.

Table 53

Patients with cognitive impairment
Correlation MMSE score - UPDRS - Intellectual impairment

MMSE-score (points)	Total number of patients with increased UPDRS-Intellectual impairment score	Number of patients with UPDRS-Intellectual impairment score			
		1	2	3	4
25	4	0	4	0	0
26	1	1	0	0	0
27	5	5	0	0	0
28	13	13	0	0	0
29	6	5	1	0	0
30	4	4	0	0	0

In the great majority of the patients there was a close relationship between the UPDRS intellectual impairment score and the MMSE score (Table 53). This correlation was also statistically on a high significant level (regression linear test $p < 0.002$). Only 4 patients had an incongruity between the MMSE score of 30 and the intellectual impairment score of 1. It is possible that the MMSE do not register all the fine changes in the cognition state at the beginning of its impairment. The age and educational level could also influence the MMSE score[158,159]. In the cohort of studied patients there were only 4 cases with a MMSE score below 26 and an intellectual impairment score of 2, among them 2 older than 80 years, and 2 younger than 75 years (Table 54).

Table 54

First neurological examination

Correlation age – MMSE score

	MMSE score			
Age group	Men	Women	Men	Women
	26–30	26–30	<26	<26
40–59	1	0	0	1
60–79	7	19	0	1
> 80	2	3	1	1

Of the patients with a MMSE score below 26 the first neurological examination and the MMSE were done in one case after 6 years, in another after 15 years and in the last 2 cases 1 year after the anamnestically reported appearance of the motor symptoms. Two of them had a low educational level.

Thus, in the studied patients the age influenced the presence of the mental impairment but less its severity. Both are mainly disease dependent.

There was found no statistical significant correlation between the intensity of motor cardinal symptoms estimated with UPDRS motor score and the MMSE score or the UPDRS intellectual impairment score (regression linear test $p < 0.05$). Moreover, there was also no statistically significant correlation between the MMSE score and the UPDRS intellectual impairment score, on one hand, and the score of tremor, rigidity, bradykinesia, postural instability, speech motor, or facial expression, separately considered, on the other hand.

Taking into consideration the above presented data, there is to assume that a mental impairment could appear already in the early stages of Parkinson's disease.

A prerequiste condition to consider a cognitive impairment as yielded by PD is to establish that at least two cardinal motor symptoms were present before the first manifestation of an intellectual impairment. According to reports of the relatives of the studied patients in whom cognitive deficits were noticed at the first neurological examination, a mild forgetfulness was observed in the months after the appearance of the cardinal motor symptoms.

Therefore, in this study a cognitive impairment was found, at the first neurological examination, in 20.67% of all patients, either alone or concurrently with mood and/or behavior disturbances, was more frequent in older persons and could affect in the onset one or more cognitive functions. None of the patients with cognitive impairment presented delusions, hallucinations or daytime sleepiness and in none of them there was a subsequently significant impairment in the non-motor activities of daily living.

2. Mood disturbance. The most frequent mood disturbance observed in the clinical picture of the PD is the depression. While Mayeux[133] mentioned that neither mania nor bipolar illness have been described in patients with PD, Ferreri F et al.[160] noticed the bipolar disorders as a rare manifestation in the PD, appearing during the on-phase, as a side effect of anticholinergic therapy, pallidotomy or deep brain stimulation. Appearing as dysthymia, as minor or major depression, the frequency of the depression was variously reported. Kremer and Starkstein[161] noticed a frequency of 5–20%, among them 18–20% major depression, Gupta and Bahtia[162] reported the presence of depression in 90% of the Parkinson patients, among them 52% with major depression, whereas Starkstein et al.[163] found in a series of 173 patients with PD in 30% a major depression, in 20% a dysthymic disorder, in 10% a minor depression and in 8% a subsyndromal depression. Other authors noticed the presence of depression in approximately half of their patients with PD[133,164,165]. The depression was found in every stage of the Parkinson's disease, but in 25% of the Parkinson patients with depression this could be observed before the onset of the motor cardinal symptoms or in the first year after the onset[133]. The pathophysiology of the depression in the PD is yet unknown. Whereas in some patients a reactive depression cannot be excluded, some authors nowadays suggest that depression in the Parkinson's disease appears secondary to changes in the function of some neurotransmitters as dopamine, serotonin, and norepinephrine[160], or to changes in central serotonergic function and neurodegeneration of specific cortical and subcortical pathways[164].

In this study the disturbance of the mood was present only as depression. Out of the 237 patients with PD 39 (16.45%) had a depression, which was present already at the first neurological examination and was less frequent than the cognitive impairment. Of the patients with depression 28 were females and 11 males with a F/M ratio = 2.54. This ratio was higher than the ratio F/M of all patients with untreated PD in this study which reached a value of 1.72 (Table 55).

Table 55

First neurological examination

Gender related frequency of depression

Age group	Number of patients	Gender	
		Male	Female
40–59	5	3	2
60–79	29	8	21
> 80	5	0	5

Actually, the depression was observed at the first examination among the 150 female patients with PD in 18.66% and among 87 male patients in 12.64% of the individuals. Thence, there is to assume that depression is a more frequent psychiatric symptom in females than in males patients with untreated PD. Baba et al.[32] found in a cohort of 1,264 individuals with PD also a significant higher frequency of depression in women than in men (35% versus 24%).

In the cohort of 237 untreated patients with PD in early stages the distribution of the depression was, unlike that of cognitive impairment, not age related. In the age group older than 80 years the percent frequency of the depression was with 14.70% nearly the same as in the group 40 to 59 years where it reached 13.88%. The frequency of the depression, alone or associated with other psychiatric symptoms, was with 17.36% somewhat higher in the age group 60 to 79 years and so accordingly to the age-related frequency of the Parkinson's disease in this study (Table 56).

Table 56

First neurological examination
Age related frequency of depression

Age group	Total number of patients	Patients with depression	Percent
40–59	36	5	13.88%
60–79	167	29	17.36%
> 80	34	5	14.70%

The depression was found at the first examination either as a sole symptom or combined with cognitive deficit and/or behavior disturbance. The number of patients with depression combined with other psychiatric symptoms was more than three times higher than that of individuals which presented only a depressive mood (Table 57).

Table 57

First neurological examination
Presence of depression

	Number of patients	
Age group	Depression Alone	Depression & other psychiatric symptoms
40–59	2	3
60–79	6	23
> 80	1	4

To estimate the intensity of the depression it was used the following rating scale:

1 = Depressed mood for up to 2 weeks, no other symptoms

2 = Persistent depressed mood for more than 2 weeks associated with low energy, tendency to a incessantly rumination, lost of interest or pleasure

3 = Persistent depressed mood associated with above mentioned symptoms and hopelessness, guilt feeling as well as with vegetative symptoms like insomnia, anorexia, weight loss

4 = Persistent depressed mood with aforementioned symptoms and suicidal thoughts or intent.

According to this scale, 20.81% of the patients with depression presented at the first examination a light depressed mood, 43.58% a minor depression and 5.12% major depression (Table 58). None of them had suicide thoughts or intent.

Table 58

First neurological examination

Severity of depression

Age group	Gender	Number of patients	Degree of depression			
			1	2	3	4
40–59	M	3	3	0	0	0
	F	2	0	2	0	0
60–79	M	8	3	5	0	0
	F	21	12	8	1	0
> 80	M	0	0	0	0	0
	F	5	2	2	1	0

Further, there was investigated the possible correlation between the severity of depression and that of the intellectual impairment.Some authors found a significant correlation between minor or major depression and severity of cognitive impairment in patients with PD[163].

In the studied 237 untreated patients with PD the majority of those with depression (58.98%) had no cognitive deficits, 35.90% a mild cognitive impairment and 5.12% a moderate one at the first neurological examination (Table 59).

Table 59

First neurological examination

Correlations depression – cognitive deficits

Age group	Depression	Degree of cognitive deficit			
	degree	0	1	2	3
40–59	I	2	1	0	0
	II	2	0	0	0
	III	0	0	0	0
60–79	I	8	7	0	0
	II	9	3	1	0
	III	0	0	1	0
>80	I	1	1	0	0
	II	1	1	0	0
	III	1	0	0	0

There was no statistically significant correlations between the intensity of the depression and the severity of the cognitive impairment (regression linear test $p<0.05$).

There was also no statistically significant correlation in these patients between the intensity of the depression and the severity of the cardinal motor symptoms, as well as between the intensity of depression and the disabilities in activities of daily living (regression linear test $p<0.05$).

These data suggest that in the early stages of Parkinson's disease:

a) The depression is less frequent than the cognitive impairment;

b) In the great majority of patients the depression manifested as a light or moderate one;

c) Commonly the depression goes along with no or only mild cognitive impairment;

d) The intensity of depression does not correlate with that of disturbances in the activities of daily living, or the severity of the cardinal motor symptoms.

3. Behavior disturbance. The behavior disturbances in patients with PD in this study was assessed according to UPDRS subscale I. The disturbances manifested as a diminution or loss of initiative. This appeared to be independently from bradykinesia or a possible bradyphrenia. The last was not observed in the early stages of Parkinson's disease. In patients with minor or major depression which presented also a reduction of initiative is questionable if the low energy observed do not influence the appearance and/or worsening of a diminished initiative .

Pluck and Brown[166] observed in Parkinson patients higher levels of apathy when compared with equally disabled osteoarthitic patients. They found that apathy in Parkinson's disease is unrelated to the disease progression but closely with cognitive impairment, and the level of apathy is rather not connected with the intensity of the depression.

Out of the 72 patients with psychiatric symptoms in this study 37 (51.38%) reported a reduction of the initiative at the first neurological examination. Only one of them presented merely a diminution of the initiative, whereas in the other 36 the reduction of initiative was associated to an impairment of the cognition and/or depression.

Table 60

Initiative reduction associated with cognition impairment and/or depression

Age group	Gender	Number of Patients	Initative reduction degree			
			1	2	3	4
40–59	M	2	2	0	0	0
	F	1	1	0	0	0
60–79	M	7	3	3	1	0
	F	17	12	5	0	0
> 80	M	2	1	1	0	0
	F	7	3	2	1	0

In the majority of individuals (62.16%) there was a slight reduction of initiative, they were more passive than before and must be sometime animated by relatives. In 29.72% there was a moderate and in 5.40% an obvious reduction of initiative (Table 60).

The gender did not influenced the frequency of the initiative reduction. Although F/M ratio regarding the initiative diminution was higher than the F/M ratio of the patients in this study, there was no significant statistical correlation between the gender and the reduction of initiative (regression linear test $p<0.05$).Although the percent frequency of the patients with diminished initiative was higher in patients older as 80 years than in those under 60 (Table 61), there was no significant statistical correlation between the age and the presence of reduced initiative in the studied individuals (regression linear test $p<0.05$).

Table 61

First neurological examination
Correlations age - reduced initiative

Age group	Percent of all patients	Percent of patients with reduced initiative
40–59	15.19%	11.11%
60–79	70.46%	14.37%
> 80	14.35%	26.47%

There was also no correlation between the intensity of initiative reduction and the severity of rigidity, or of bradykinesia (regression linear test $p<0.05$).

Autonomic dysfunctions

Among the signs and symptoms of the Parkinson's disease there are also such which represent a dysfunction of the autonomic nervous system. In the last two decades the interest of clinical research was focused on the presence, frequency and moment of appearance of these symptoms in PD. It was postulated that some of them could appear already in early stages of PD and even before the cardinal motor symptoms become evident.

Because of that there was looked for to the presence and the moment of appearance of autonomic disturbances in this cohort of patients with untreated Parkinson's disease.

In the clinical picture of the PD were delineated various symptoms of autonomic nervous system disturbances including: gastrointestinal, urogenital, cardiovascular, thermoregulatory, pupillary and epidermal glands (sebaceous) dysfunctions and also sleep abnormalities[167].

1. Gastrointestinal dysfunction. The presence of gastrointestinal disorders in Parkinson's disease, although already mentioned by James Parkinson in his monography in 1817, became of interest for neurologists and researchers only in the past twenty years.

As gastrointestinal symptoms in Parkinson's disease are considered: salivary excess, dysphagia, gastroparesis, small intestine dysmotility, colon dysmotility, anorectal dysfunction and weight loss[168,169,170,171,172,173,174,175]. In the majority of cases these symptoms were described on the basis of clinical and/or laboratory investigations done in patients with treated PD in various Hoehn &Yahr clinical stages. The number of untreated parkinsonian patients with gastrointestinal (GI) symptoms was small, the majority in early clinical stages, and all gastrointestinal symptoms comparable to those of treated subjects, except the defecatory dysfunction, which was more frequent in treated patients[169].

Gastrointestinal symptoms could be asymptomatically present already in early stages of Parkinson's disease[172,176]. Nevertheless, it was of interest to assess the moment when these dysfunctions become clinically evident, while only then they could be important for daily practice. The presence of GI symptoms in this study was assessed exclusively on clinical basis, i e. interview of the patients and relatives and detailed clinical examination at the first contact with the patient.

Salivary excess. Out of 237 untreated patients 29 or 12.23% reported an excess of salivation. Among them 25 had a slight (only night-time drooling) and 4 a moderately excessive salivation according to UPDRS item 6. However there must be mentioned that a night-time drooling without the presence of at least two cardinal motor symptoms cannot be considered as parkinsonian symptom. A night-time drooling can be observed also in persons sleeping with open mouth. Among the 29 patients with excess of saliva there were 18 women and 11 men with a F/M ratio of 1.63, which was not significant different from the F/M ratio of 1.72 in this study. There was also no statistical significant correlation between the drooling and gender (regression linear test $p < 0.05$).

Furthermore, there was no correlation between age at the clinical onset of the disease and the appearance of salivary excess. The frequency of abnormal salivation in these individuals did not increase along the age (Table 62). The correlation was not statistical significant (regression linear test $p < 0.05$).

The duration of the disease from the anamnestically reported clinical onset up to the first neurological examination, too, did not influence the frequency of excessive salivation or it intensity (regression linear test p<0.05).

Table 62

First neurological examination

Correlation age – salivary excess - dysphagia

Age group	Percent of all patients	Percent frequency of excessive salivation	Percent frequency of swallow difficulties
40–59	15.19%	16.66%	13.88%
60–79	70.46%	11.97%	8.98%
> 80	14.35%	11.76%	2.94%

In the studied patients, in early stages of PD, the frequency of excessive salivation seemed not to be influenced by the intensity of the motor symptoms. There was no statistically significant correlation between the salivary excess and UPDRS motor score (regression linear test p<0.05). Nonetheless, that seems to be a correlation between the localization of the motor symptoms (uni- or bilateral) and the presence of abnormal salivation. Actually, all patients with salivary excess were in clinical stages 2 or 2.5 after Hoehn & Yahr (Fig.9).

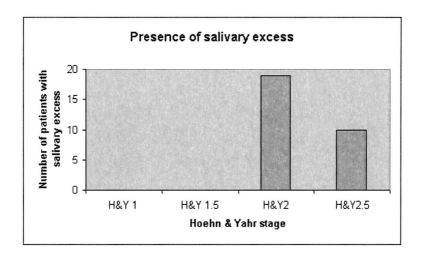

Fig. 9 First neurological examination. Correlation of salivary excess with Hoehn & Yahr stages

Taking into consideration that the salivary excess is not yield by an overactivity of the salivary glands but a result of chewing and swallowing disturbances[173,177], there could be possible that the excessive salivation is in fact the first manifestation of the dysphagia.

Dysphagia. According to some authors[168] dysphagia occurs in many patients with PD and is usually asymptomatic. Pfeiffer[173] reported swallowing difficulty in 30–82% and abnormalites in barium swallow testing in 75–97% of subjects with PD.

Out of the studied 237 patients 21 (8.86%) complained at the first medical interview about choking. In all these individuals the choking was reported as rare and subsequently assessed with 1 point on the UPDRS item 8. Among the subjects with swallow disturbances were 9 men and 12 women with a F/M ratio of 1.3. Thus, the swallow disturbances were somewhat more frequent in men (10.34%) than in women (8%).

The age-related frequency of the swallow dysfunction was in the age group 40 to 59 years higher than in the age group 60 to 79, and obviously higher than in patients older than 80 years where the choking was reported only by 2,94% individuals (Table 62). The frequency of swallow disturbances in the studied patients did not go along with progression in age and did not statistically correlate with the age (regression linear test $p<0.05$).

In 76.19% of individuals the swallow disturbances was noticed in the first two years after the clinical onset and only in 19% more than 3 years after the reported onset. It was no statistically significant correlation between the frequency of swallow difficulties and disease duration (regression linear test $p<0.05$).

The intensity of motor symptoms had no influence on the frequency of dysphagia in the early stages of PD. There were no statistical significant differences regarding the UPDRS motor score between individuals with and without dysphagia in this study (one-way ANOVA $p<0.05$). The presence of dysphagia correlated rather with the bilaterality of the motor symptoms. None of the patients with hemiparkinsonism (Hoehn & Yahr stage 1) complained of swallow disturbances, only 2 were in stage 1.5 Hoehn&Yahr, and the great majority of individuals with swallow abnormality (90.50%) were in stage 2 or 2.5 Hoehn&Yahr at the first neurological examination (Fig. 10).

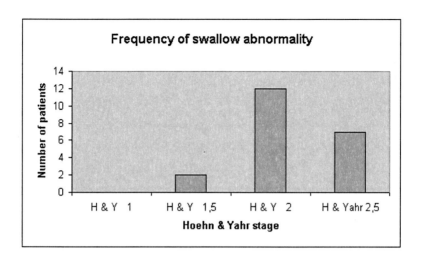

Fig. 10 First neurological examination. Correlation swallow abnormality - Hoehn & Yahr stage**s**

In patients with bilateral symptoms and postural instability (Hoehn &Yahr stage 2.5) the percent frequency of swallow difficulties was with 12.28% higher than those in individuals without postural instability (Hoehn &Yahr stage 2) which had a frequency of 7.18%.

Therefore, the dysphagia becomes symptomatically already in the early stages of PD, especially in patients with bilateral and axial motor symptoms and its frequency seems to be dependent neither from the intensity of motor symptoms nor from the time elapsed between the onset of symptoms and the moment of first neurological examination, but rather from the bilaterality of the motor symptoms.

Gastroparesis. The presence of gastroparesis in PD was delineated particularly in the past decade[172,174,178]. As symptoms were described the following: early satiety, anorexia, abdominal fullness, bloating,nausea and vomiting. Gastroparesis was noticed in the moderate stages (Hoehn & Yahr 2.5 and 3) as well as in the mild stages (Hoehn&Yahr 1–2) and its prevalence was not significantly different between these two groups[172]. According to some authors[175] the gastroparesis is associated with the severity of motor impairment, whereas others[172] found no relationship between delayed gastric emptying and other clinical features of PD.

In the studied population of 237 untreated patients in early stages of PD no signs or symptoms of gastroparesis were reported, especially neither anorexia nor nausea or vomiting. It is possible that other symptoms of gastroparesis were not mentioned by the patients since they considered not to be in connection with their neurological complaints and hence not mentioned at the interview with the neurologist. However the identification of gastroparesis already in the early stages of Parkinson's disease remains important also for the diagnosis of PD, since it could influence the L-Dopa Test and eventually falsify the result.

Constipation. Constipation and defecation difficulties are common symptoms in PD. According to Pfeiffer[173] the defecatory dysfunction is the more prevalent form of bowel dysfunction in PD. The constipation is considered as present when there are less than 3 bowel movements weekly, whereas symptoms of defecation difficulties are regarded excessive straining by defecation accompanied by pain and sensation of incomplete evacuation. The frequency of constipation reported in the literature varies between 20 and 70% according to authors[168,179]. The defecation dsyfunction in patients with PD estimated by anorectal manometry reached a high frequency up to 60%[170,179], and was also observed in early stages of the disease.

Out of the 237 patients in this study 28, or 12%, mentioned an occasional or more frequent constipation, which in some individuals appeared as chronic and in few even before the first motor symptoms of the PD.

In the last years the constipation is regarded, by some, as a well-documented premotor symptom in PD, along with hyposmia, depression and rapid eye movement sleep behavior disorder (RBD)[180,181].

Taking into consideration also the neuropathological data which document the presence of Lewy bodies not only in the central and peripheral autonomic nervous system, but also in the enteric nervous system (Auerbach's and Meissner's plexuses)[167, 182,183,184,185], there would be of great interest to investigate how many patients complaining on chronic constipation have parkinsonian symptoms, or would those become in the following years. Since there are yet no biological markers to identify the Parkinson's disease in its preclinical stage, probably only a naturalistic approach would clarify if there is a causal relationship between a chronic constipation and a later appearance of Parkinson's disease. This presume a neurological follow up of persons with chronic constipation over several years.

Weight loss in the studied patients exclusively correlated with PD was reported neither by patients nor by relatives.

2. Sexual dysfunction. A decreased libido is a common delineated symptom in PD. A frequency up to 83% for men and 84% for women was reported in the literature. A frequency up to 40% was reported by persons older than 70 years in this cohort of untreated parkinsonian patients. Nonetheless, that remains questionable to what extent the sexual dysfunction, because of the frequent comorbidity especially in this age group, could be attribute only to Parkinson's disease. The same is valid for erectile dysfunction in men, which was also noticed in this study.

3. Urinary dysfunction. Although urinary symptoms were already mentioned by James Parkinson in 1817, only in the XXth century they attracted the attention of the clinicians. Nowadays, lower tract urinary symptoms, either irritative or obstructive, are considered common symptoms in PD. Various authors reported the presence of urinary symptoms in the clinical picture of the PD [186,187,188,189,190,191,192]. The frequency of the irritative symptoms varies between 53%-83% and that of obstructive symptoms between 23-36%.

Considering the presence of lower tract urinary symptoms in the clinical picture of the patients with Parkinson's disease, either irritative or obstructive, it is necessary above all, with regard to the age-related comorbidity, to exclude other illness with similar symptoms (internal, urological).

Out of the 237 studied patients only 8 patients reported lower tract urinary symptoms which in absence of other illness could be correlated with the presence of PD. Some other patients with mild parkinsonian symptomatic reported at the first neurological examination also urinary symptoms, which were attributed to already known urological or gynecological diseases.

Hence, in the daily practice, before lower tract urinary symptoms are assigned to the Parkinson's disease other illness should be excluded.

4. Cardiovascular dysfunction. In the past two decades various authors investigated the autonomic cardiovascular disturbances in the Parkinson's disease. Two clinical symptoms of cardiovascular autonomic dysfunction were delineated:

a) orthostatic hypotension,

b) reduced heart rate variability(HRV) [193,194,195,196,197,198,199,200,201,202,203,204,205] .

a). *Orthostatic hypotension* is a common manifestation in PD with a prevalence up to 58.2%, and can be present symptomatically but also with higher frequency asymptomatically[200]. Whereas some authors noticed the orthostatic hypotension (OH) in more advanced stages of PD, and correlated its presence with the severity and duration of the disease and with the dosis of dopaminergic medication, others found no significant differences in the functions of the autonomic nervous system between the levodopa treated and the untreated patients[194,197]. Some studies consider OH as an early finding in PD, and hypothesize that cardiac noradrenergic denervation and decreased baroreflex cardiovagal dysfunction could appear early in the course of the disease [206,207,208].

The presence of orthostatic hypotension in the patients included in this study was investigated by using a detailed personal interview, in which special attention was directed to the presence of dizziness, visual disturbances and falls, and by measuring the blood pressure and heart rate supine and standing. Signs and symptoms of orthostatic dysregulation of the blood pressure in the early stages of PD were neither mentioned nor observed in the studied patients. Some elderly females accused at the first neurological examination a dizziness position change-dependent, but there was found no blood pressure or heart rate drop by position changing from supine in standing.

b) *Reduced heart rate variability*, also a common cardiac symptom in patients with PD, is caused by the dysfunction of the cardiovascular autonomic system.

In the up to now works there is assumed that the reducing of the heart rate variability (HRV) is the result both of sympathetic and parasympathetic cardiac autonomic dysfunction[194,195,196,209,210,211,212,213].

A consecutive investigation was done in 56 patients with Parkinson's disease,not included in this study, to estimate the presence of HRV changes. The individuals with diabetes mellitus, myocardial infarction, cardial rhythm disturbances or cerebral infarct in the anamnesis were excluded. Out of the 56 patients 40 were treated with L-Dopa alone, or combined with other antiparkinsonian medication (dopamine-agonists and/or amantadine, selegiline, rasagiline) while the other 16 were yet untreated patients. There were 37 women and 19 men with a F/M ratio of 1.94. The age range was 54 to 93 years with a mean age of 72.96 (SD± 6.89) and a statistical median age of 74 years.

Table 63

Patients with 24-hour ECG

Age group	Number of patients	M	F	HRV attenuated	(%)	HRV normal	(%)
40–59	6	2	4	2	33.33%	4	66.66%
60–79	37	16	22	14	37.84%	23	62.16%
> 80	13	2	11	6	46%	7	54%

The percent frequency of patients with reduced HRV increased with the age (Table 63), but there was no statistically significant correlation between age and presence of diminished HRV in these patients (regression linear test $p<0.05$). There was also no statistical significant differences concerning the age between the patients with attenuated and those with normal HRV (one-way ANOVA $p<0.05$).

The disease duration range was 1-22 years with a mean value of 9.82 years (SD±3.84) and a statistical median of 8 years. Out of the 56 patients with 24-hour ECG 46.5% had a disease duration of 6 to 10 years, 19.64% a disease duration of 11 to 15, and 16% a disease duration up to 5 years (Fig.11).

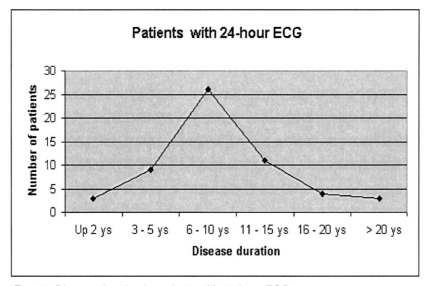

Fig. 11 Disease duration in patients with 24-hour ECG

97

The peak frequency of normal HRV was in patients with disease duration 6-10 years (Fig.12)

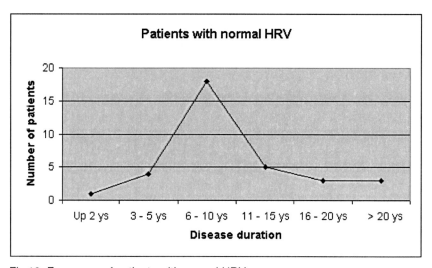

Fig.12 Frequency of patients with normal HRV

Although in a few patients an attenuated HRV was found after a disease duration of up to 5 years, respectively 16 to 20 years, the great majority of the patients with reduced HRV (86.35%) had a disease duration from 5 up to 15 years with a peak also in the disease duration group of 6 to 10 years (Fig. 13).

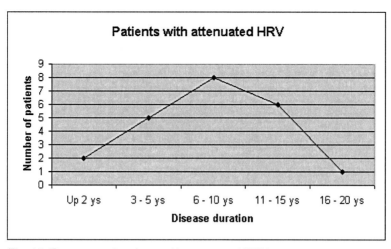

Fig. 13 Frequency of patients with attenuated HRV

There was no statistically significant correlation between the duration of the disease and the frequency of reduced HRV in these patients (regression linear test $p < 0.05$), as well as no statistical significant difference concerning the disease duration between the patients with and those without attenuated HRV in this group (one-way ANOVA $p < 0.05$).

Furthermore, neither the severity of the cardinal motor symptoms estimated with the UPDRS motor score nor the degree of disability estimated with the Hoehn & Yahr scale influenced the appearance of reduced HRV. There was no statistically significant correlation between the frequency of reduced HRV and the intensity of the cardinal motor symptoms, as well as no statistically significant correlation between the frequency of attenuated HRV and the clinical stage after Hoehn&Yahr (regression linear test $p < 0.05$). A third of untreated parkinsonian patients presented at the first neurological examination also an attenuated HRV. However the number of investigated patients is too low to draw a conclusion on the prevalence of reduced HTV in the early stages of untreated PD.

Therefore, it is to assume that in many patients with Parkinson's disease an attenuated HRV, as a manifestation of cardiac autonomic dysfunction, could be present. It is neither age nor gender dependent, has no relationship with disease duration, severity of motor symptoms, or degree of disability according to Hoehn and Yahr scale. An attenuated heart rate variability appears already in the early stages of Parkinson's disease, both with regard to the clinical stages after Hoehn & Yahr and to the disease duration.

However, not all patients with PD have clinically orthostatic hypotension or reduced heart rate variability on ECG, although some of them have a reduced cardiac 123I MIBG uptake, reflecting a cardiac sympathetic dysfunction[214], which could occur early in PD[215].

The question why in some patients despite the presence of neuroimaging and cardiac testing data for a cardiac denervation, clinical symptoms like orthostatic hypotension or heart rate variability are missing is not yet answered.

5 .Thermoregulation disturbance. A dysfunction of the thermoregulation in patients with PD was already mentioned by Charcot and later by Gowers in 1888[216]. Some patients complained about a discomfort for heat, while some others about an abnormal sensation of cold. However, as some authors found, the patients with PD, unlike the MSA patients, had a 24-hour rhythm of body core temperature comparable to controls[217].

In the patients of this study, all in early stages of PD, there was anamnestically no reports of abnormal feelings of heat or cold.

An excessive sweating as manifestation of the thermoregulation dysfunction was also reported in patients with PD[218,219,220,221,222,223,224]. The sweat dysfunction in PD is considered to be a product of functional disturbances of sympathetic postganglionic fibers[221,222]. In some patients authors had noticed a higher perspiration in the upper part of the body (the forehead, chest and forearm) and a diminished one on the dorsal parts of hand and foot than in control subjects. According to some authors there is significant correlation between the increase of perspiration and the severity of the disease[223]. In the early stages of PD there was observed only a minor sudomotor disturbance rendered evident by the impairment of TRH (thyrotropin-releasing hormone) - induced sympathetic response which did not increase the sweat rate in patients with PD as seen in controls[220].

Out of the 237 studied patients with untreated PD only 3 mentioned a hyperhidrosis among other parkinsonian signs and symptoms at the first neurological examination. They were 3 females: 2 in the age group 60 to 79 and 1 in the age group >80 years. The excessive perspiration in these patients involved mainly the head, trunk and axilla. These data are based on the statements of the patients and on the first clinical examination.

6 . Respiratory disturbance. In the past three decades the respiratory disturbances in PD got the attention of various authors and specialists. It is now wide accepted that the Parkinson's disease affects the respiratory tract and that at all levels [225].

Already Hoehn and Yahr[12] incriminated the high frequency of pneumonia as cause of death in Parkinson patients as compared to the general population. The death due to pneumonia was not dependent upon the age of the patient or duration of the disease. Afterwards many authors could confirm the high frequency of pneumonia as cause of death in patients with Parkinson's disease[226, 227,228,229,230,231]. As studies of the past twenty years showed, the upper airway obstruction is the most frequent respiratory disturbance and its subclinical presence could be found in up to nearly 50% of the investigated patients with Parkinson's disease, whereas the restrictive pulmonary dysfunction was less frequent[232,233,234,235,236,237]. This concerned patients in moderate to severe disease stage (stage III to V on the Hoehn & Yahr scale) and was explained by the involvement of the respiratory musculature in the parkinsonian process. Very few of them had also a clinical symptomatic.

In this study on 237 untreated parkinsonian patients clinical signs and symptoms of respiratory tract dysfunction were not observed

7. Epidermal glands (sebaceous) dysfunction. A dysfunction of sebaceous glands was for long ago noticed in the Parkinson's disease. The hyperscretion of the sebaceous glands of the face causes the seborrhoea that gives to the face skin a shine look known as "facies oleosa." This symptom observed in the middle and especially advanced stages of the PD appeared usually in connection with amimia.

In the studied patients, who were all in the early stages of PD, no seborrhoea of the face was observed.

Sensorial symptoms

Olfactory dysfunction

In the past three decades numerous studies demonstrated disturbances of the olfactory function in patients with PD[238,239,240,241,242,243,244,245,246,247,248,249]. Accordingly, up to 90% of the patients with PD had a deficit in smell identification. However, hyposmia could be observed also in other neurological and psychiatric diseases (dementia of the Alzheimer type, Huntington's chorea, Korsakoff's psychosis, craniocerebral traumata etc.), endocrine disease (diabetes), and others.

In 60 patients with PD the smell identification was tested with the Sniffin'
Sticks. Out of them 18 were patients in early stages of PD included in this study. The
others were patients with Parkinson's disease under therapy with antiparkinsonian
drugs, patients with essential tremor and patients with Lewy-Body dementia (Table
64).

Table 64

Patients undergoing smell identification test

	Number of patients	Smell test		
		Normal	Hyposmia	Anosmia
Pat. with untreated PD	18	2	12	4
Pat. with treated PD	37	0	18	19
Pat. with Lewy bodydementia	3	0	1	2
Pat. with essential tremor	2	0	2	0

The patients with essential tremor presented too a mild extrapyramidal syndrom, but
the SPECT with ^{123}I-FP-CIT showed no pathological changes of the dopamine
transporters.

All but 2 patients of the 55 patients with untreated and treated PD tested had a
deficit in the smell identification test. Although a smell identification deficit was found
nearly in up to 90% of patients with untreated PD, this cannot be considered as
pathognomonic for the Parkinson's disease, since, as already mentioned, other
diseases too can cause a smell dysfunction.

As authors already pointed out[240,241], the olfactory dysfunction in parkinsonism
is unrelated to neurologic signs, disease stage, duration, or therapie with
antiparkinsonian drugs. The pathological correlate of olfactory dysfunction in PD
seems to be the presence of neuronal loss in anterior olfactory nucleus (AON), and
the presence of Lewy bodies in the olfactory bulb and tract and also in the
rhinencephalon (amygdala, hypothalamus, cingulum, hippocampus and
frontotemporal cortex)[242]. However other authors found a 100% increase of
dopaminergic cells in the olfactory bulb of patients with PD, which could explain the

hyposmia in Parkinson's disease (dopamine inhibits the olfactory transmisson in the olfactory glomeruli)[250].

Anyway, the presence of a smell dysfunction could be regarded as forerunner of the Parkinson's disease only when all other causes were excluded and the presence of parkinsonian symptoms could be proved concurrently or before long.

Sensitive symptoms

Along with the well-known motor symptoms some patients with Parkinson's disease mentioned at the first neurological examination also disturbances of the epicritic sensitivity namely: paresthesia, dysesthesia and pain.

In the studied patients with untreated PD the frequency of such symptoms was below 10%. In some patients sensory symptoms, especially pain, appeared already in the preclinical stage of the PD and was a reason to see a physician. Six of the untreated patients with PD in this group reported cervical or shoulder pain as a reason to consult a physician. Since no orthopedic objective symptoms were found, the patients consulted a neurologist who diagnosed the Parkinson's disease. Other epicritic sensitivity symptoms, like dysesthesia and paresthesia, were rather mentioned after the diagnosis was settled, during the follow-up.

These symptoms could be brought in connection with the PD when, on the one hand, they were inconstant and variable with respect to their localization and, on the other hand, no other causes explaining the complaints could be found.

Correlations clinical stages Hoehn & Yahr - UPDRS score

The nowadays widely accepted and used scale of Hoehn and Yahr[12] is, as the authors said, "an arbitrary scale based on the level of clinical disability." Accordingly, they described a five-level scale taking into account the anatomical extension of the symptoms for the first stages of the scale and the severity of body disability for the last stages. On the UPDRS (1997) the Hoehn & Yahr scale has 8 levels of disability (0, 1, 1.5, 2, 2.5, 3, 4, 5) correlated with the extension of the symptoms for the first stages and with the disability severity for the last stages. The wide use of scales in estimating the extension and intensity of the symptoms of Parkinson syndrome in the last 20 years made it necessary, also for practical purposes, to investigate the correlations between the clinical stages of the Hoehn & Yahr scale and the scores of the UPDRS, the most frequent scale used nowadays.

In fact, whereas a patient with PD could remain several years in the same H & Y clinical stage, the intensity of symptoms, when estimated accordingly to UPDRS, could change and this could be important for assessing the prognosis as well as the subsequent therapy.

Of the 237 studied patients with untreated PD only 7 were in the stage 1 and 7 in the stage 1.5 on the Hoehn & Yahr scale. The majority were in stage 2 (151 patients or 63.71%) and in stage 2.5 (72 or 30.37%). There were no patients in higher stages on the Hoehn & Year scale.The low number of individuals with unilateral PD in this cohort of patients is in accord with the observations of Hoehn & Yahr[12].

The high frequency of the bilateral parkinsonian symptomatic found at the first neurological examination could be explained by the fact that these patients went to see a physician several months up to 1 to 2 years or later after the noticed onset of the signs and symptoms of the Parkinson's disease.

Investigating the correlations between the total score and the motor score of UPDRS, on the one hand, and the clinical stages of Hoehn & Yahr scale, on the other hand, there was found a close relationship between the scores of UPDRS and the clinical stages on the Hoehn & Yahr scale. The total score and the motor score of the UPDRS increased concurrently with the levels of the Hoehn & Yahr scale (Table 65).

Table 65

First neurological examination

Correlations Hoehn & Yahr stages – UPDRS score

Hoehn & Yahr stage	Number of patients	UPDRS score	
		T – score	M – score
1	7	11.70 (± 4.81)	8.64 (± 2.44)
1.5	7	18.28 (± 4.81)	11.57 (± 3.08)
2	151	21.89 (±7.28)	17.10 (± 5.49)
2.5	72	31.76 (±9.70)	23.95 (± 7.34)

Legend

T – score = Subscale I + Subscale II + Subscale III score

M – score = Subscale III score

The mean UPDRS T-score increased along with severity of clinical disability (Fig.14).

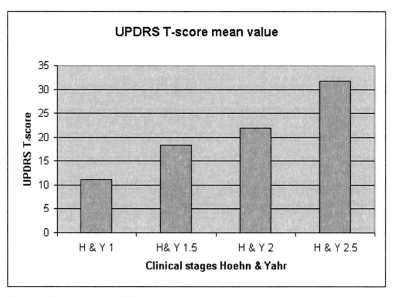

Fig.14 Correlations UPDRS T-score mean value - clinical stages Hoehn & Yahr

There were statistically significant differences in the UPDRS T-scores between the patients in H & Y clinical stage 1 when compared with those in clinical stage 1.5, and especially between subjects in stages 1 and 1.5 and those in stage 2, as well as between individuals in stage 2 and those in stage 2.5 (one-way ANOVA p<0.05).

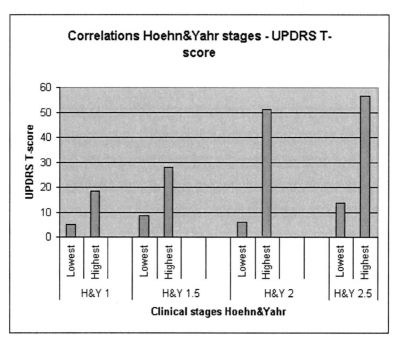

Fig.15 First neurological examination. Correlations clinical stages H & Y – UPDRS
T-score

The lowest and the highest UPDRS T-scores, as well as the UPDRS motor scores, in the studied patients, were different along the clinical stages Hoehn & Yahr. So, in the H & Y stage 1 the lowest and the highest UPDRS T-scores were 5 and 18.5 points respectively, whereas in the H & Y stage 2.5 the lowest T-score was 13.5 and the highest 56.5 points (Fig. 15).

These data showed that in the same clinical stage Hoehn & Yahr the UPDRS T-scores as well as the motor scores could be different interindividual, i.e. in the same clinical stage are subjects with various UPDRS scores. It is well known that individuals with Parkinson's disease once they reached a certain Hoehn&Yahr clinical stage could remain in the same stage for several or more years[12], whereas the number and especially the intensity of symptoms increase along the time.

Therefore, the Hoehn&Yahr scale, at least in the early stages of PD, reflects rather the anatomical spread of the disease and not the number or severity of the motor and non-motor symptoms.

Thence, to estimate the severity of the Parkinson's disease there must be taken into consideration several features: the anatomical extension of the motor symptoms (unilateral, unilateral + axial, bilateral), the intensity of the symptoms, the presence of signs and symptoms indicating a disturbance of the autonomous nervous system, the presence of a mental impairment, and the degree of disability.

Although the UPDRS in the present form does not yet reflect some symptoms and only insufficiently others, is still closer to an allround assessment of the symptoms and allows a better estimation of the disease severity on a certain moment.

For that reasons, and to better estimate the severity, prognosis, and efficacy of the therapy it is useful to assess the severity of the Parkinson's disease on the basis of Hoehn and Yahr scale and of UPDRS score.

Diagnosis of Parkinson's disease

The diagnosis algorithmus of the PD undergoes 2 phases:

1. The diagnosis of the Parkinson syndrome (PS)

2. The diagnosis of Parkinson's disease (PD), i.e. idiopathic Parkinson syndrome.

1. Diagnosis of Parkinson syndrome (PS) is primary a clinical one. Whereas the presence of a sole parkinsonian symptom like mild bradykinesia, or shuffling gait, or slight rigidity, was, and is still considered a normal aging manifestation in older people, especially in persons of the " third age" (older than 75 years), the concurrent presence of at least 2 main parkinsonian motor symptoms (bradykinesia, tremor, rigidity, postural instability), found incidental in otherwise normal considered older individuals could raise diagnostical questions. Community-based studies in persons without dementia older than 65 years noticed the presence of mild parkinsonian signs (MPS), with a prevalence ranging from 2.3% in several European communities[251] to 7.2% in a community in Brazil[19] to 16.1%[20] and 25.1%[21] in communities in USA.

These data point out that only a small part of otherwise neurologically normal considered old people have parkinsonian signs or symptoms and, thus, that can not be excluded the possibility that these symptoms are rather manifestations of an underlying disease than of normal aging .

Although there are definite clinical criteria proposed to diagnose parkinsonism[252,253], this could be still a challenge, since, on the one hand, the prevalence of PS is increasing with the age, as seen in this study and as reported by other authors[251], and, on the other hand, as community-dwelling studies showed, older people and their relatives because of the mild symptomatic are not aware, or considered them normal aging manifestations.

In the studied cohort of 237 untreated patients with PD 18.56% had at the first neurological examination 2 and 81.44% 3 or 4 cardinal motor symptoms.

Out of the 237 subjects 36.28% reported anamnestically the appearance of at least 2 cardinal motor symptoms as the clinical onset of the disease, whereas 63.72% reported only one symptom. The great majority of the last group accused tremor as first manifestation. Analyzing the reported disease history of these patients that gets obviously that the bradykinesia and the rigidity are at the beginning ignored, whereas a tremulous hand was promptly noticed and caused the consult of a physician. Moreover, the patients with tremor in the anamnesis could better set the appearance date and first localization of this symptom than the others who had as first symptom bradykinesia or rigidity.

According to the UK Parkinson's disease Society Brain Bank[252], the clinical diagnosis of parkinsonism can be put when at least 2 of the following 4 cardinal motor symptoms are present at the same time in the clinical picture and one of them is bradykinesia:

- Bradykinesia,

- Muscular rigidity,

- 4-6 Hz rest tremor

- Postural instability not caused by primary visual, vestibular, cerebellar, or proprioceptive dysfunction.

Of the 237 patients in this study 215 (90.71%) presented at the first neurological examination bradykinesia and 233 (98.31%) rigidity, beside other motor cardinal symptoms. Moreover, not all patients with tremor had a resting tremor but also/or a postural/action tremor.

Thus, the absence of bradykinesia, or the presence of postural/action tremor instead of resting tremor at the first neurological examination do not exclude the diagnosis of parkinsonism. The data of this study showed that to diagnose Parkinson syndrome there is necessary the presence of at least 2 cardinal motor symptoms, one of them bradykinesia or rigidity. The absence of bradykinesia by concurrent presence of rigidity, rest tremor and/or postural instability at the first examination cannot exclude the diagnosis of PS.

None of the cardinal motor symptoms taken alone allows the clinical diagnosis of Parkinson syndrome. In one patient, not included in this study, with a primary restless legs syndrome and a mild to moderate rigidity without bradykinesia, tremor, or postural instability, the SPECT with ^{123}I-FP-CIT was normal.The clinical picture remained unchanged during a follow-up of more than 9 years.

In this phase the diagnosis of idiopathic Parkinson syndrome is basically a possible diagnosis.

2. Diagnosis of Parkinson's disease (PD) is a probable diagnosis, does not be restricted on clinical signs and symptoms, and requires also some ancillary investigations to exclude other causes of PS.

The diagnosis of probable PD in the studied patients underwent 3 stages:

a) Extensive anamnestical interview of the patient and his relatives,

b) Detailed neurological examination,

c) Ancillary investigations.

a) The extensive anamnestical interview aimed not only to identify the appearance of the cardinal motor symptoms at the clinical onset of the disease, but also the sequence of their appearance, the first anatomical localization (uni- or bilateral), the subsequent spread of symptoms, the eventual presence of severe cognitive deficits and of autonomic dysfunctions, especially orthostatic hypotension and miction disturbances. Furthermore, the personal interview had as objective to clarify if the patient took a medication which could cause extrapyramidal signs and symptoms.

b) The detailed neurological examination was done not only according to UPDRS, but it was investigated in detail also all other anatomical systems of central, peripheral and autonomous nervous system.

Following criteria was stated as clinical criteria of probable Parkinson's disease in early stages:

- the exclusive presence of extrapyramidal signs in the clinical picture,

- unilateral onset when proved (anamnestically or clinically),

- asymmetric intensity of the extrapyramidal signs, only with reference to the anatomical localization of the symptoms,

- absence of dementia.

The presence of postural/action tremor instead of resting tremor did not exclude a probable idiopathic Parkinson syndrome when the tremor was accompanied by at least two other cardinal motor symptoms. The postural instability was commonly at the first neurological examination. In none of these patients there was a severe postural instability manifested as a frequent tendency to spontaneously lose of body balance and falling.

c) Ancillary investigations were mainly aimed to support the delimitation of probable PD from the secondary or atypical Parkinson syndromes.
All patients in this study unterwent a cranial computer tomography or a cranial MRI examination. These investigations allowed largely to exclude a secondary PS, as well as an atypical form of it.

None of the patients in this study became a L-Dopa test, or dopamine agonists on trial basis because they refused medication.

Postmortem studies on the putamen and caudate nucleus in patients with Parkinsons's disease showed a nearly complete depletion of dopamine in putamen and a reduction in caudate nucleus[263,264]. Going out from these data, studies in vivo with radionuclide substances binding to pre- or postsynaptic dopamine receptors tried to estimate the presence and quantity of dopamine in striatum.
In the past 18 years numerous authors attempted to support the diagnosis of probable PD by PET and SPECT investigations with radionuclide substances[254,255,256,257,258,259,260,261,262]. These studies found in patients with idiopathic Parkinson's disease (PD) a significantly lower uptake of these radioligands in striatum, especially in putamen, when compared with healthy control persons.

Other studies using also radiotracers as biomarker had as purpose to distinguish between the idiopathic Parkinson's disease and other parkinsonian syndromes either as part of atypical Parkison syndrome like multiple-system atrophy or progressive supranuclear palsy, or as a result of drugs (neuroleptics, calcium channel blockers, antiemetic, antivertigo, etc.), cerebral vascular disturbances or psychogenic origin[261,265,266,267,268]. In all parkinsonian syndromes other than the idiopathic one independently of their origins, the concentration of the radioligands in the striatum was reported either as normal or in a concentration that was below that of healthy persons but above that found in patients with Parkinson's disease. Generally that is considered that the patients with drug-induced Parkinson syndrome, with vascular parkinsonismus or psychogen PS have normal concentration values of radioligands binding to dopamine transporters of the presynaptic terminals of dopaminergic neurons in striatum.

The estimation of Dopamine transporters (DAT) in striatum with [123]I-ß-CIT or ^{123}I-FP-CIT and SPECT has, according to some authors, a sensitivity up to 90-100% and a specificity of up to 98%, although according to others[262] in older patients (aged over 55 years) the specificity reached only 68.5%. In a group of 35 patients, but 1 not included in this study, in whom an investigation with ^{123}I-FP-CIT and SPECT was done, it was found for Parkison's disease a sensitivity of 64% and a specificity of 36%.

However, nowadays there remains the question how useful is the imaging of DAT in the daily clinical practice. The Parkinson's Disease Society appreciates that approximately 5-25% of patients with suspected parkinsonism may require ^{123}I-FP-CIT imaging[269]. Other authors[262] concluded that [123]I-ß-CIT may not be as useful in the clinical practice as previously believed, or SPECT scanning may not be useful in differentiating PD from other parkinsonian syndromes[270]. Ravina B, Eidelberg D et al.[271] reviewing the use of the radiotracers in the imaging of the nigrostriatal dopaminergic system and the evidences supporting the use of four radiotracers as biomarkers in PD concluded that, although measuring relevant biologic processes, they do not measure the number or density of dopaminergic neurons and "current evidence does not support the use of imaging as a diagnostic tool in clinical practice or as a surrogate endpoint in clinical trials."

Therefore the diagnosis of probable PD remains yet a diagnosis " per exclusionem."

Since in some patients an atypical PS (MSA-P, PSP-P) can begin with the same clinical picture as that of PD and only years later other symptoms of atypical PS appear, the diagnosis of PD must again and again be checked.

Course of Parkinson's disease in the early stages

The follow-up of the patients with PD without antiparkinsonian medication in this study allowed some observations on the natural course of Parkinson's disease.

It is well known that the onset of the clinical symptoms is inconspicuous, their appearance and development at the beginning lingering.

There is generally assumed that Parkinson's disease has, according to different authors, a preclinical period of 5 up to 15–20 years, which is very poor in signs referring to parkinsonian syndrome. In the past two decades some autonomic and sensorial signs like constipation, hyposmia, were proposed as precursors of motor symptoms in Parkinson's disease. However these signs were found, with various frequency, only concurrently with the motor symptoms. There are yet no prospective studies going out from non-motor symptoms, which could prove that these ones are in a causal and temporal connexion with the motor symptoms of parkinsonian syndrome.

In this study there was found in the anamnesis of patients no clues of the presence of non-motor symptoms preceding the appearance of the cardinal motor symptoms.

There was also of interest to see the manner the motor symptoms appeared in the clinical picture: concurrently or one after the other.

At the first neurological examination out of the 151 patients which claimed anamnestically a sole cardinal symptom none had only one, but already 2, 3 or 4 motor cardinal symptoms. The time elapsed between the appearance of the parkinsonian symptoms in patients with anamnestical one cardinal symptom and the first neurological examination was up to 1 year in 76.15% of the patients, up to 3 years in 13.25% and in the rest of 10.60% more than 4 up to 10 years.

Thus, in the great majority of these patients after 1 year already 2, 3 or 4 cardinal motor symptoms were present. This allows two presumptions: either the parkinsonian motor symptoms appeared concurrently, but the patients noticed only one of them, or they appeared in a short succession, one after another. From the anamnesis it was not possible to find out how the motor symptoms appeared and if there was a certain pattern in their appeerence.

However, taking into consideration all patients in this study, the number of patients with 2 cardinal symptoms decreased proportional more than those of patients with 3 and 4 cardinal motor symptoms when the first neurological examination was done later (Fig.16).

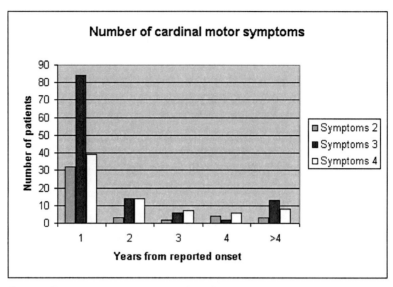

Fig. 16 First neurological examination. Correlations number of cardinal motor symptoms – duration in years from reported onset

That is possible that the number of motor cardinal symptoms, in some patients, increased along the time elapsed from the anamnestically reported clinical onset to the first neurological examination, and as a result the frequency of 3 or 4 cardinal symptoms in the clinical picture was higher than that one of 2 cardinal symptoms.

Evolution of the parkinsonian symptomatic

Of the 237 studied patients 137 were examined once again after 10-12 weeks. In these patients both the number of the motor cardinal symptoms and their intensity remained unchanged. Because of that the evolution of the pakinsonian symptomatic was assessed only on the 100 patients which were followed more than 3 months, some up to 86 months, after the first neurological examination.

Presence of the cardinal motor symptoms.
Out of the 100 patients which could be followed more than 3 months presented at the first neurological examination: 49 individuals 3 cardinal motor symptoms, 36 persons 4, and 15 others 2 cardinal motor symptoms (Fig.17).

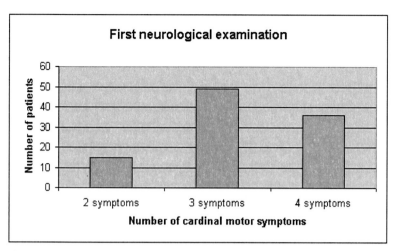

Fig. 17 Patients with a follow-up of more than 3 months

The motor cardinal symptoms were found in various combinations, among them the most frequent was the rigidity followed by bradykinesia, postural instability and tremor (Table 66).

Table 66

Follow up more than 3 months
First neurological examination
Combinations of the motor cardinal symptoms

Motor symptoms	Number of patients
Bradykinesia + Rigidity	11
Rigidity + Tremor	2
Rigidity + Postural instability	2
Bradykinesia + Rigidity + Tremor	15
Bradykinesia + Rigidity + Postural instability	29
Bradykinesia + Tremor + Postural instability	1
Rigidity + Tremor + Postural instability	4
Bradykinesia + Rigidity + Tremor + Postural instability	36

The great majority of these patients was examined neurologically every third month during a follow-up of at least 3 up to 86 months. The 36 individuals, but two, who presented all four motor cardinal symptoms already at the first neurological examination, retained these symptoms along the entire follow-up time. Out of the other 64 patients with 2 or 3 motor cardinal symptoms 24 (37.5%) presented additionally at the following neurological examinations one more motor cardinal symptoms (Table 67).

Table 67

Follow up more than 3 months

Later appeared motor cardinal symptoms

First neurological examination	Following neurological examinations	Number of patients	Duration up to change
Bradykinesia + Rigidity	Bradykinesia + Rigidity+ Postural instability	8	3–13 months
Rigidity + Tremor	Rigidity + Tremor + Bradykinese	2	3–4 months
Rigidity + Postural instability	Rigidity + Postural instability + Bradykinesia	2	3–4 months
Bradykinesia + Rigidity + Tremor	Bradykinesia + Rigidity+ Tremor+ Postural instability	5	4–7 months
Bradykinesia+ Rigidity+ Postural instability	Bradykinesia+ Rigidity+ Postural instability + Tremor	4	3–8 months
Rigidity + Tremor + Postural instability	Rigidity + Tremor + Postural instability+ Bradykinesia	3	4–7 months

The number of motor cardinal symptoms in these patients remained, after the appearance of another cardinal symptom, unchanged until the end point of the study. The endpoint was either the moment when the patient did no more appear in the practice, or when the subject became an antiparkinsonian medication. Thus, the endpoint could be other than the appearence moment of an additional motor cardinal symptom, and different for every patient.

Out of the 100 patients observed more than 3 months the number of those with 2 motor cardinal symptoms decreased with 28.57%, that with 3 motor symptoms increased with 11.52%, and the number of individuals with 4 motor cardinal symptoms was lower with 6% at the last neurological examination when compared with the first one (Fig.18).

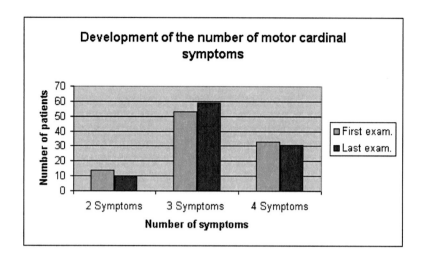

Fig.18 Changes of the number of main motor symptoms during the follow-up

These data suggest that in the early stages of Parkinson's disease the development of the parkinsonian symptomatic is still in course and the main motor symptoms could also appear one after the another. It suggest also the possibility that these symptoms could appear in the same manner at the onset of the disease before the first neurological examination but were not noticed by the patients. If confirmed, these observations are important to better understand the pathophysiology of the PD, as well as to develop neuroprotective agents.

Furthermore, the art of appearance of the motor symptoms could be regarded as possible predictive factor concerning the progression of the Parkinson's disease along with the development of the severity of these symptoms. The longer a patient remains with the same number and same intensity of cardinal motor symptoms the better could be the prognosis.

Course of cardinal motor symptoms intensity .

The intensity and development of the motor cardinal symptoms was assessed according to the UPDRS motor score.

At the last neurological examination of 100 patients, which were followed up more than 3 months, bradykinesia was present in 100, rigidity also in 100, postural instability in 80, resting tremor in 34, and postural/action tremor in 50 individuals. Whereas in some patients the severity of these symptoms remained unchanged at the last neurological examination when compared with the first one, there were in others differences in the intensity of motor cardinal symptoms (Table 68).

Table 68

Follow-up more than 3 months

Intensity course of cardinal motor symptoms

Symptoms	Number of Patients	E > B	B > E	E = B
Bradykinesia	100	55	36	9
Rigidity	100	52	32	16
Postural instability	80	20	23	37
Resting Tremor	33	6	19	8
Postural/action tremor	50	14	20	16

Legend   E = Last neurological examination

B = First neurological examination

Bradykinesia. The intensity of bradykinesia was assessed by comparing the bradykinesia scores accordingly to UPDRS at the last to those at the first neurological examination. As bradykinesia score was considered the sum of finger taps, hand movement, rapid alternating hand movement and leg agility scores. The score of each item varied from 0 to 4.

Of the 100 patients which were followed from 3 to 86 months, 57 patients had an increased bradykinesia score at the end of the follow-up, while in 34 the score was less and in 9 the same as at the first neurological examination. Both the increase and the decrease of the bradykinesia score was not a linear process along the follow-up, since the score varied somewhat from one examination to the other, but the trend to increase or decrease remained. In the both groups the bradykinesia score differences between the last and first neurological examination were statistically significant (one-way ANOVA $p < 0.05$).

The changes in the intensity of bradykinesia during the follow-up was influenced neither by age nor gender, nor by the duration of the disease estimated from the anamnestically reported clinical onset up to the last neurological examination. There was no statistical significant correlation between age, gender and disease duration and the severity of bradykinesia in the studied patients (regression linear test $p<0.05$). The course of bradykinesia, as such, during the follow-up evolved independently from that of rigidity. There was also no statistical significant correlations between the course of these two symptoms i.e. bradykinesia and rigidity (regression linear test $p<0.05$).

With regard to the aggravation of the bradykinesia a worsening of its score was found in 63% of patients already in the first year, and in 80% in the first 2 years after the PD was diagnosed. The worsening trend of the bradykinesia from the first to the next or over next neurological examination could possible also serve as predictor for the development of the disease.

Rigidity. Among the 100 followed-up individuals 16 had the same intensity of rigidity of the neck and extremities muscles at the last as at the first neurological examination. In all other patients the intensity of the rigidity was different. In 52 (52%) of the cases the rigidity score was at last examination higher, and in other 32 (32%) lower than at the first examination. However, in the patients with a lower rigidity score at the end of the follow-up the differences in rigidity score between last and first examination were not significant, while in the group with ,a higher rigidity score at the last neurological examination the differences were statistically highly significant (one-way ANOVA $p<0.05$).

During the follow-up in many patients could be noticed intraindividual changes of the rigidity with regard to the anatomical distribution and the severity. The intensity of the rigidity could change when one side of the body was compared with the opposite, or the rigidity of the neck or arm muscles when compared with that of the legs.

The course of the rigidity during the observation time was not influenced by age, gender, or disease duration from the reported clinical onset until the end of the study. There was no statistical significant correlations between the changes of rigidity and age, gender and disease duration (regression linear test $p<0.05$). The changes of the intensity of bradykinesia during the follow-up did not influence the changes of the rigidity.

Tremor. The intensity of the tremor was estimated exclusively on the basis of own neurological observation during an examination of the patient from 30-45 minutes in on-state.

The criteria to appreciate the tremor intensity were:

- the extension of the affected anatomic segment (finger, hand, arm, foot, leg),
- the duration of the tremor presence, depending also from the possibility of the patient to suppress intermittently the tremor, or from the necessity to divert the patient to favor the appearance of the tremor,
- the amplitude of the tremor.

On the basis of these criteria the following scale was used to estimate the resting tremor of the hand:

0 = absent;

1 = mild, affects mainly the thumb or all finger, small in amplitude, intermitent, or mostly observed on diverted patients,

2 = moderate, the tremor is longer time persistent, could affect the entire hand, nevertheless can be still suppressed by the patient and the amplitude is small,

3 = evident, the tremor is persistent for the time of examination, affects the whole hand, can still be suppressed for short time by carrying out another task and the amplitude is larger,

4 = marked, the tremor is persistent all the time of examination, affects not only the hand but also the forearm or the whole arm, cannot be suppressed intentionally or by carrying out another task and the amplitude is great.

The emotional state of the patient must also be taken into consideration when assessing the intensity of the tremor, since the simple presence of examiner could augment its intensity.

Out of the followed-up cohort of 100 patients 37 had no tremor. Of the other 63 observed patients 13 had a resting tremor, 30 a postural/action and 20 at the same time a resting tremor and a postural/action one. At the first neurological examination were already present the resting tremor in 28 individuals and the postural/action tremor in 45. Later, during the follow-up, the tremor at rest appeared in other 5, and the postural/action tremor also in other 5 patients.

Both the resting tremor and the action/postural tremor score varied in many patients also intraindividually during the follow-up. The intensity of the tremor was changed in the majority of the patients when the last neurological examination was compared with the first one. Of 33 patients who manifested a tremor at rest alone or together with an action/postural tremor the tremor end score was in 19 patients lower, in 6 higher and in 8 the same as at the first neurological examination. The differences were statistically significant (one-way ANOVA p<0.05). In the group of the 30 patients with postural/action tremor alone in 12 the score was at the last neurological examination lower, in 7 was higher, and in 11 was the same as at the first neurological examination. In those patients with postural/action tremor and score changes the differences in the tremor score between the last and first neurological examination were also statistical significant (one-way ANOVA p<0.05).

Furthermore, in many patients during the follow-up the tremor intensity could change from one neurological examination to the next.

The changes in tremor intensity total score as well as the changes in presence and intensity of the resting tremor, or postural/action during the follow-up was influenced neither by age nor by gender or duration of the follow-up. There was no statistically significant correlations between the changes in presence and intensity of the resting tremor, or of the postural/action tremor, or tremor total score and the age, the gender or the disease duration up to the endpoint of the study (regression linear test p<0.05).

Postural instability. Of the 100 patients followed up more than 3 months 67 were women and 33 men with a female/male ratio (F/M ratio) of 2.03. Twenty of them had no postural instability during the follow-up. Among them were 10 men and 10 women (Table 69). Eleven of them were followed up to 1 year and the other 9 between 2 to 6 years. Eight of other 80 individuals with postural instability at the last neurological examination presented no postural imbalance at the first examination. In other 38 individuals the intensity of postural imbalance was at the last neurological examination the same as at the first one, in 19 more severe than at the first examination and in 23 less severe. Besides, changes in the intensity of the postural disbalance could be observed also in the same patient during the clinical observation independently from the severity of the postural instability at the last neurological examination.

Although the frequency of postural instability seemed to increase in women patients (Table 69) there was no significant statistical correlation between gender and the changes of postural disbalance severity during the obsevation time (regression linear test p<0.05).

Thence, in 10% of the patients with postural imbalance this appeared during the follow-up. This proves that in some individuals cardinal motor symptoms could appear later in the disease progress.

Table 69

Follow-up more than 3 months

Correlations postural instability - gender

Postural instability	Number of patients	Men	Women	F/M Ratio
No postural instability	20	10 (50%)	10 (50%)	1
		Postural instability		
B = E	38	13 (34.21%)	25 (65.79%)	1.92
E > B	19	3 (15.78%)	16 (84.21%)	5.33
B > E	23	7 (30.44%)	16 (69.56%)	2.28

Legend

B = First neurological examination

E = Last neurological examination

F/M Ratio = Female/Male Ratio

To assess the influence of the age on the course of the postural instability and on its severity, there was investigated the correlations between age and changes in the intensity score of postural disbalance.

The age of the patients did not influence the moment of appearance of postural instability and the course of its intensity (Table 70). There was no statistical significant correlations between age and presence and changes of postural imbalance intensity during the follow-up (regression linear Test $p < 0.05\%$). There were also no statistical significant differences regarding the age between the patients in whom the intensity of postural instability was increased and those in whom the intensity was decreased or remained the same at the last neurological examination compared to the first one (one-way ANOVA $p < 0.05$).

Table 70

Follow-up more than 3 months

Correlations age – postural instability

		Age groups					
		40–59		60–79		> 80	
		Duration of follow - up in months					
Intensity score	Number of Patients	3–12	> 12	3–12	> 12	3–12	>12
E > B	19	3	0	11	5	0	0
B > E	23	1	0	10	8	1	3
B = E	38	3	2	21	6	3	3
No postural instability	20	3	1	7	7	1	1

Legend

B = First neurological examination

E = Last neurological examination

To determine if the disease duration could influence the intensity of the postural instability in the early stages of the illness, the changes of the postural imbalance were correlated with the disease duration from the reported clinical onset up to the study endpoint.

There were only very few changes in the severity of the postural disbalance at the endpoint of the study when compared with first neurological examination (Table 71).

There was found no significant statistical correlation between the disease duration and the frequency of postural imbalance in these patients (regression linear test $p<0.05$). There were also no statistically significant differences with regard to the changes in the postural disbalance severity at the last neurological examination when compared with the first one (one-way ANOVA $p<0.05$).

Table 71

Follow-up more than 3 months

Correlations disease duration – postural stability

	Normal	Postural Instability			
		Degree of severity			
		1	2	2.5	3
First neurological examination	29	26	15	30	0
Last neurological examination	28	28	17	26	1

Further, there was investigated if the other motor symptoms could influence the postural imbalance during the course of the disease. Whereas the changes of the rigidity intensity and of the tremor did not influence the postural disbalance, there was found a close connection between the changes of the bradykinesia intensity and those of postural instability. There was a high significant statistical correlation between the course of bradykinesia and the changes of postural instability (regression linear test p=0.005).

At the last neurological examination, there was also a statistically significant correlation with some other axial motor symptoms, namely with dysarthrophonia and arising from chair, but not with hypomimia (regression linear test p<0.05).

Accordingly, it is to assume that the presence and development of the postural imbalance could be influenced by other motor symptoms, especially by bradykinesia, whereas age, gender and disease duration has no influence.

As already above presented, the postural instability takes an important place in the classification of the clinical stages according to Hoehn and Yahr scale.

Because of that, there was also looked for the correlations between the changes in the severity of postural instability and the clinical stages after Hoehn and Yahr in the patients followed up more than three months.

Table 72

Correlations Hoehn & Yahr stages – postural instability

Last against first neurological examination

H &Y stages	Number of patients	No post. instability at last examination	Postural instability		
			E = B	E > B	B > E
1	1	1	0	0	0
1.5	3	2	0	0	1
2	66	25	15	19	7
2.5	30	0	20	1	9

Legend

B = First neurological examination

E = Last neurological examination

Out of the 100 studied patients only one was in Hoehn&Yahr stage 1 and had no postural instability. Two of 3 individuals with unilateral and axial symptomatic (Horhn&Yahr stage 1.5) had also no postural instability according to above delineated scale, and 1 a moderated instability, which improved during the follow-up. Of the 96 patients with bilateral parkinsonian symptomatic 66 was considered in stage 2 and 30 in stage 2.5 on the modified Hoehn and Yahr scale. During the follow-up, 25 of the 66 patients in stage 2 Hoehn&Yahr had no postural instability, while in the other 41 the intensity of postural imbalance was at the last examination in 15 individuals unchanged, in 19 worsened, and in 7 improved. Of the 30 patients in Hoehn&Yahr stage 2.5, which had at the first neurological examination an evident postural instability, in 20 it remained unchanged, in 9 improved, and in 1 worsened (Table 72).

The intensity of the postural imbalance could also change in the same patient during the follow-up, from one neurological examination to the next one. The more severe degree of the postural disbalance once appeared remained in the majority of patients unchanged until the last examination, whereas the mild or moderate could improve in some individuals.

Therefore, in the early stages of PD the development of the postural instability could go along with the course of bradykinesia and some other axial motor symptoms (dysarthrophonia and arising from chair), its intensity is fluctuating, not dependent from the duration of disease, could influence the degree of disability, and consequently the classification in one or other clinical stage on the Hoehn and Yahr scale.

Course of axial motor symptoms

Camptocormia. Of the 100 patients who could be followed more than 3 up to 86 months 29 presented camptocormia with different intensities. In the other 71 the posture was normal.

Among the patients with camptocormia whose intensity was mild to moderate according to above delineated scale, the intensity remained in 7 unchanged, in 14 improved, and in 8 was either a new appearance (in 6), or worsened when the score at the last neurological examination was compared with that at the first one. The gender did not influence the changes in the intensity of camptocormia. The age, too, had no influence of the course of camptocormia intensity during the follow-up (Table 73).

Table 73

Follow-up more than 3 months
Correlations camptocormia intensity – age

		Age group					
		40–59 ys		60–79 ys		> 80 ys	
Camptocormia intensity	Number of patients	Follow up duration in months					
		3–12	> 12	3–12	>12	3–12	>12
E = B	7	0	0	3	2	1	1
E > B	8	0	0	2	4	2	0
B > E	14	0	0	6	3	1	4

Legend

B = First neurological examination

E = Last neurological examination

There was no statistically significant differences regarding the age of patients between the groups of individuals in whom the intensity of camptocormia was at the last neurological examination the same, increased or diminished when compared with the first neurological examination (one-way ANOVA $p<0.05$).

There was no statistically significant correlation between the disease duration estimated since the reported clinical onset until the first, respectively the last neurological examination, and the appearance and intensity of camptocormia (regression linear test $p<0.05$). There was also no statistically significant difference with respect to disease duration when the score intensity of camptocormia at the last examination was compared with the intensity of the camptocormia score at the first one, but only in a group of 6 patients in whom camptocormia appeared during the follow-up (one-way ANOVA $p<0.05$).

On the basis of these data there is to presume that in the early stages of PD, i.e in the first 1-2 years after the reported clinical onset, in the great majority of patients the appearance and intensity of camptocormia is not dependent from the disease duration.

The intensity of camptocormia was in this cohort of patients also not dependent from the rigidity respectively bradykinesia score at the last neurological examination. There was no statistical significant correlation between the intensity score of the camptocormia and that of the rigidity, respectively of the bradykinesia at the end of the study (regression linear test $p<0.05$). Nevertheless, when compared the course of camptocormia intensity with that of rigidity respectively bradykinesia expressed in the score difference between last and first neurological examination the changes of the camptocormia severity correlated on a statistical significant level with those of rigidity but not with those of bradykinesia severity (regression linear test $p<0.05$).

Therefore, these data suggest that in the early stages of PD the development of the abnormal posture correlated with that of the rigidity, whereas the course of the postural instability correlated with that of the bradykinesia.

There was a close correlation between the presence and intensity of the camptocormia and that of some other axial motor symptoms as dysarthrophonia, hypomimia and arising from chair. Whereas at the first neurological examination there was a significant statistical correlation only between the presence and intensity of the camptocormia and that of the hypomimia, at the last neurological examination the correlation between severity of the camptocormia and that of other axial motor symptoms (dysarthrophonia, hypomimia, arising from chair) was statistically high significant (regression linear test p<0.05).

Dysarthrophonia. Speech disturbances were present in 71 out of the 100 patients followed up more than 3 months. Among the individuals with dysarthrophonia there were 47 women and 24 men and so nearly twice more frequent in females (F/M Ratio: 1.96). The monotonous, low voice appeared in 31% of the patients for the first time during the follow-up, after the first neurological examination, in 65% of them in the first 12 months.

The age influenced the appearance of voice disturbance but not its development in the early stages of PD. In fact, out of the 71 patients with voice disturbances only 4.22% were younger than 60, whereas in the group of those without dysarthrophonia the percent under 60 reached 31% (Table 74).

There was a high significant statistical correlation between age and presence of voice disturbances at the end of the study (regression linear test p<0.05) but no statistically significant differences between the group of individuals with no changes in the intensity of dysarthrophonia at the end of the study and the groups with worsening or improvement of speech disturbances (one-way ANOVA p<0.05).

Table 74

Follow-up more than 3 months
Correlations dysarthrophonia – age

Dysarthrophonia intensity	Number of patients	Age group					
		40–59 ys.		60–79 ys.		> 80 ys.	
		Follow-up duration in months					
		3–12	>12	3–12	>12	3–12	>12
E = B	41	2	0	17	15	2	5
E > B	23	0	1	12	6	3	1
B > E	7	0	0	2	4	0	1
No dysarthrophonia	29	7	2	18	2	0	0

Legend

E = Last neurological examination

B = First neurological examination

Hence, that is to assume that in the early of PD the age could influence the moment of appearance but not the severity of dysarthrophonia.

The duration of the disease, too, estimated since the clinical onset until the last neurological examination, had no influence on the intensity of voice disturbances. In this group of patients there was no statistical significant correlation between the duration of disease and the appearance and severity of dysarthophonia (regression linear test $p<0.05$), as were no statistical significant differences regarding the disease duration between those with no changes of dysarthrophonia intensity and those with worsening of it at the end of the study (one-way ANOVA $p<0.05$).

The course of speech disturbances were also not concurrently with the development of the rigidity as well as of the bradykinesia score in patients with a follow-up of more than 3 months. There were, on one hand, no statistical significant correlation between the course of the dysarthrophonia intensity and that of the rigidity, respectively of the bradykinesia (regression linear test $p<0.05$) and, on the other hand, no statistical significant differences regarding the rigidity, respectively bradykinesia scores between individuals with no changes in the intensity of dysarthrophonia and those with worsening of it at the end of the study (one-way ANOVA p<0.05).

Facial expression. The hypomimia was present in 30% out of the 100 patients followed up more than 3 months, and so, obviously, not so frequent as the dysarthrophonia which reached 71%. The frequency of the hypomimia in female patients was four times higher than in men at the first neurological examination and thrice at the last one. However, there was no statistically significant correlation between the gender and the frequency of hypomimia at the first as well as at the last neurological examination, and also no influence of the gender on the changes of the hypomimia during the follow-up (regression linear test p<0.05).

In the patients followed up more than 3 months the frequency of the hypomimia appeared to be influenced by age. None of the patients younger than 60 presented a hypomimia at the first as well as at the last neurological examination (Table 75).

Table 75

Follow-up more than 3 months

Correlations hypomimia – age

		Age group					
		40–59 ys.		60–79 ys.		> 80 ys.	
Hypomimia intensity	Number of patients	Follow up duration in months					
		3–12	>12	3–12	>12	3–12	<12
E = B	15	0	0	4	6	2	3
E > B	16	0	0	8	5	2	1
B > E	9	0	0	5	2	0	2
No hypomimia	60	9	3	33	13	1	1

Legend

E = Last neurological examination

B = First neurological examination

Actually, there was a statistically high significant correlation between the age and the presence of hypomimia in this group of patients (regression linear test

131

p<0.05). However, the severity of the hypomimia estimated according to UPDRS were not influenced by the age. There was no statistical significant correlation between the age and the changes of the hypomimia during the follow-up (regression linear test $p<0.05$) as well as no statistical significant difference with regard to the age between the patients with higher and those with lower hypomimia score (one-way ANOVA $p<0.05$).

In the early stages of PD the disease duration, estimated from the reported clinical onset until the last neurological examination, does not seem to influence the appearance and intensity of the hypomimia. There was no statistical significant correlation between the duration of the disease and the presence of the hypomimia at the last neurological examination (regression linear test $p<0.05$). There were also no statistical significant differences with respect to disease duration, between the group of patients with worsened hypomimia at the last examination and those with improved or no changed hypomimia intensity (one-way ANOVA $p<0.05$).

In this study there was found no connection between the intensity of the limbs rigidity or that of the extremities bradykinesia and the appearance and severity of hypomimia in the early stages of PD. There was no statistical significant correlation between the presence and intensity of the rigidity, respectively of the bradykinesia of the limbs, and the appearance and intensity of the hypomimia (regression linear test $p<0.05$).

The presence of the hypomimia correlated statistically on a high significant level with that of the speech motor disturbances not only at the first neurological examination but also at the last one (regression linear test $p<0.05$). However, the changes in the severity of hypomimia during the follow-up were to a large extent independent from those in the intensity of dysarthrophonia. In fact, there were no statistical significant correlations between the changes of the speech disturbance intensity and those of the hypomimia intensity during the observation time (regression-linear test $p<0.05$).

Arising from chair. Difficulties in arising from chair were present in 43 of the 100 patients followed up more than 3 months. Out of the patients with difficulties in arising from chair were more women than men. However there was neither at the first nor at the last neurological examination statistical significant correlations between the gender and the frequency of the difficulties in arising from chair (regression linear test $p<0.05$). The gender had also no statistically significant influence on the changes of arising from chair difficulties during the follow-up (regression linear test p<0.05). In 27.90% of the patients with difficulties in arising from chair these appeared during the course of the disease, whereas in other 41.86% these difficulties were no more present at the last examination.

The great majority of patients with difficulties in arising from chair was older than 60 (Table 76). However there was no statistically significant correlation between the presence of difficulties in arising from chair and the age of patients observed more than 3 months (regression linear test p<0.05).

Moreover, there were no statistically significant differences regarding the age between individuals with no changes and those with increased difficulties in arising from chair at the last neurological examination when compared with the first one (one-way ANOVA p<0.05).

Table 76

Follow-up more than 3 months

Correlations arising from chair – age

		Age group					
		40–59 ys.		60–79 ys.		>80 ys.	
Arising from chair difficulties	Number of patients	Follow up duration in months					
		3–12	>12	3–12	>12	3–12	>12
E = B	7	0	0	3	1	2	1
E > B	17	0	0	6	8	1	2
B > E	20	2	0	9	6	0	3

Legend
E = Last neurological examination
B = First neurological examination

Therefore, neither the gender nor the age had influence on the frequency and variability of arising from chair difficulties in these patients.

In the followed-up patients, in early stages of PD, the disease duration, estimated from the reported clinical onset until the end of the study, did not influence the presence of arising from chair difficulties. There was no statistical significant correlation between disease duration and the presence of difficulties in arising from chair at the last neurological examination (regression linear test p<0.05).

It seems that the presence and intensity of the bradykinesia could influence the appearance and severity of the arising from chair difficulties. Actually, in the studied patients there was a statistically significant correlation between the presence and intensity of bradykinesia, on the one hand, and the presence of arising from chair difficulties, on the other hand (regression linear test p<0.05), and statistically significant differences regarding the bradykinesia scores when patients with difficulties in arising from chair were compared with those without such difficulties (one-side ANOVA p<0.05).

There was also observed certain correlations between the presence of some axial motor symptoms. So, there was a statistical significant correlation between the presence of the hypomimia and the arising from chair difficulties, as well as between the last ones and the presence of dysarthrophonia but not between the intensity of these symptoms (regression linear test p<0.05).

Course of non-motor symptoms
Psychiatric symptoms.

Cognitive impairment. The intellectual status was estimated on the basis of the anamnesis, reports of the relatives and psychiatric exploration at every neurological examination during the clinical observation of these patients. The estimation of the cognition impairment was made according to UPDRS item 1. The patients with intellectual impairment unterwent also a MMS examination.

Of the studied 100 patients only 18 had a light impairment of cognition. In 16 individuals the cognitive impairement was present already at the first neurological examination as a mild forgetfulness, and in the other 2 it appeared during the follow-up. Of the 18 individuals there were 15 women and 3 men. Although the frequency of intellectual impairment was obviously higher in females, there was no statistically significant correlation between gender and cognition impairment either at the beginning of the follow-up or at the last neurological examination (regression linear Test p<0.05). The course of the intellectual status too was not influenced by gender. The gender was not a predictor for the appearance and development of the intellectual impairment.

Not the same was the influence of the age.

Table 77

Follow-up more than 3 months
Cognitive impairment

		Age group					
		40–59 ys.		60–79 ys.		> 80 ys.	
Cognitive impairment	Number of patients	Follow up in years					
		<1 y	>1 y	<1 y	>1 y	<1 y	>1 y
E = B	7	0	0	3	1	1	2
E > B	5	0	0	2	1	0	2
B > E	6	0	0	2	4	0	0

Legend

E = Last neurological examination

B = First neurological examination

The cognitive impairment was present only in patients older than 60 years (Table77) and its frequency increased concurrently with the age. So, in the age group 40 to 59 the frequency of cognitive impairment was 0%, in the age group 60 to 79 reached 14.47%, and in the group older than 80 years increased to 41.66%. In all of the individuals with light intellectual impairment there was no influence on the activities of daily living. There was found a high significant statistical correlation between age and frequency of intellectual impairment at the first, as well as at the last neurological examination (regression linear test $p<0.05$), and also between age and course of intellectual impairment (regression linear test $p<0.05$). So far, the age could be considered as a predictor for the appearance of intellectual impairment in PD.

Of the 16 patients with light cognition impairment 4 reached at the first neurological examination 30 points in the MMSE and 12 had 28 or 29 points. There was no differences in the MMSE values between the group of patients with no changes in the intensity of cognition impairment and those with improvement or worsening of the cognition impairment during the follow-up.

It is possible that in the early stages of the PD the MMSE do not reflect the fine changes in the mental state of the patients with PD. Because of that, when the anamnesis, the reports of the relatives, and the psychiatric examination reveal clues for an eventual presence of a cognition impairment the use of finer neuropsychological tests could possibly bring more information about the first changes of the cognition state in these patients.

In the followed up patients there was no correlation between the disease duration from the clinical onset up to the first respectively last neurological examination and the appearance of intellectual impairment (regression linear test $p < 0.05$).

There was also no correlation between the intensity and course of the motor cardinal symptoms and the development of the cognition impairment in the studied individuals. Actually, all the 18 patients with cognition impairment presented at the end of the clinical follow-up a worsening on the UPDRS motor score, which was statistically significant and in the great majority of the patients also clinically relevant, whereas the cognitive impairment remained unchanged, improved and only in 3 out of 18 worsened.

The clinical anatomical localization of the cardinal motor symptoms did not influenced the presence of intellectual impairment. There was no statistical significant correlation between the localization of the motor cardinal symptoms (unilateral, unilateral & axial, bilateral) and the intellectual impairment (regression linear test $p < 0.05$).

Therefore, on the basis of these data that is to assume that a light cognitive impairment could be manifest already in the early stages of the PD, i.e. in the first 2 years after the reported clinical onset, and its appearance and course correlate mainly with the age, but not with gender and anatomical localization or intensity of the cardinal motor symptoms.

Depression. The presence of the depression was established on the basis of the anamnesis, reports of the relatives and psychiatric exploration done at the first examination and after that at every clinical investigation of the patients. The intensity of depression was estimated according to UPDRS subscale I item 3.

Out of the 100 followed-up patients 24% manifested at the first neurological examination or later during the observation signs and symptoms of depression, a percentage close to that reported also by other authors[133], only 2 of them had symptoms of a major depression roughly corresponding to the level 3 of the UPDRS subscale I item 3. In one of these two patients the major depression was present already at the first neurological examination but no more found at the last examination after 86 months, whereas in the other one the depression developed during the follow-up and reached the level 3 of the item 3 at the final examination after 57 months.

Out of the 24 patients with depression in 6 subjects that was present with the same intensity at the final neurological examination. Of other 18 individuals in 9 the depression appeared during the follow-up, in 7 was no more present and in 2 somewhat worsened at the last neurological examination (Table 78).

Table 78

Follow-up more than 3 months

Correlation depression – age – follow-up duration

		Age group					
		40–59 ys.		60–79 ys.		> 80 ys.	
Depression	Number of patients	Follow - up duration in years					
		<1 y	>1 y	<1 y	>1 y	<1 y	>1y
E = B	6	1	0	2	2	0	1
E > B	11	1	1	5	4	0	0
B > E	7	0	0	2	3	1	1

Legend

E = Last neurological examination

B = First neurological examination

The frequency of the depression in patients observed more than 3 months was higher in women.

However there was no statistical significant correlation between the course of depression and gender (regression linear test $p<0.05$).

There was also no statistically significant correlation between the course of the depression and the age of patients, or the duration of the follow-up (regression linear test $p<0.05$). Neither the age nor the gender, nor the duration of the follow-up (i.e. of the disease duration) were statistical predictors for the progress of the depression.

The course of this symptom during the follow-up did correlated neither with the course of the rigidity nor with that of the tremor, bradykinesia, or postural instability score (regression linear test $p<0.05$).

As could be observed on the followed up patients, in the early stages of the Parkinson's disease signs and symptoms of depression could appear also after the first neurological examination, and could have a various course. In the great majority of the observed patients this mood disturbance was manifested as minor depression. The presence and course of depression were not correlated with the cause and intensity of the motor cardinal symptoms, and not related to the severity of physical disability as seen by other authors[272,273].

Motivation/Initiative. The presence and severity of this symptom was estimated according to UPDRS subscale I item 4. Out of the 100 patients followed up more than 3 months 21 presented a reduced motivation/initiative. In none of these it appeared as a sole psychiatric manifestation, but accompanying the depression and/or the cognitive impairment. At the last neurological examination there was a statistical significant correlation of the reduced motivation/initiative with the presence of the depression, as well as with the presence of the cognitive impairment (regression linear test $p<0.05$).

Of the 21 individuals with reduced motivation/initiative there were 4 men and 17 women. However, at the last neurological examination there was no statistically significant correlation between the frequency of the reduced initiative and the gender (regression linear test $p<0.05$). The gender was not a statistical predictor regarding the frequency of reduced motivation/initiative in these patients.

The frequency of reduced motivation/initiative was not influenced by the age. Of the 100 patients followed up more than 3 months the percent frequency of motivation/initiative diminution reached in the age group 40 to 59 years 25%, in the group 60 to 79 years 19.73% and in the individuals older than 80 25%. There was no statistical significant correlation between reduced motivation/initiative at the end point of the study and the age (regression linear Test $p<0.05$).

In these patients, there was also no correlation between the duration of the observation and the frequency of motivation/initiative disturbances (Table 79).

Table 79

Follow-up more than 3 months
Correlations motivation/initiative – age – follow-up duration

		Age group					
		40–59 ys.		60–79 ys.		> 80 ys.	
Initiative disturbance	Number of Patients	Follow - up duration in years					
		<1 y	>1 y	<1 y	>1 y	<1 y	>1 y
E = B	2	1	0	0	1	0	0
E > B	12	1	1	4	5	0	1
B > E	7	0	0	3	2	1	1

Further, there was no statistical significant correlation between the severity of reduced motivation/initiative, on one hand, and the intensity of tremor, rigidity, bradykinesia, or postural instability, on the other hand (regression linear test p<0.05). Thus, in these patients, in the early stages of PD, the course of cardinal motor symptoms did not influenced the disturbances of motivation/initiative.

Autonomic disturbances

Out of the 100 patients followed up more than 3 months the great majority, namely 88, could be observed up to 3 years, 9 up to 5 years, 2 up to 6 years and 1 up to 7 years after the first neurological examination. None of these patients reported signs and in none were found symptoms of gastrointestinal, urinary, autonomic cardiovascular, thermoregulation or upper and lower airways dysfunction at the first as well as at the following neurological examinations. However in none of these patients were done investigations to look for the possible presence of such yet asymptomatic dysfunction. Even when in some patients of this population one or other dysfunction of the autonomic nervous system should be subclinically present, it became not manifest during the following up.

Course of parkinsonian disability

The degree of disability in the early stages of PD was estimated according to the modified Hoehn & Yahr staging as presented in UPDRS (1997).

Of the 100 patients followed up more than 3 months, 80 were at the last neurological examination in the same Hoehn & Yahr clinical stage as at the first examination, 9 in a higher, and 11 in a lower stage. The age range in patients with changed Hoehn&Yahr stage at the end of the study varied between 54-87 years, and in those without change between 44-91 years. There were no statistically significant differences with respect to the age between individuals with higher and those with lower stage Hoehn &Yahr at the last examination (one-way ANOVA $p<0.05$).

In the studied patients the age did not influenced the severity of parkinsonian disability in the early stages of PD.

The disease duration range in this group of patients was 1 to 11 years (Fig.19).

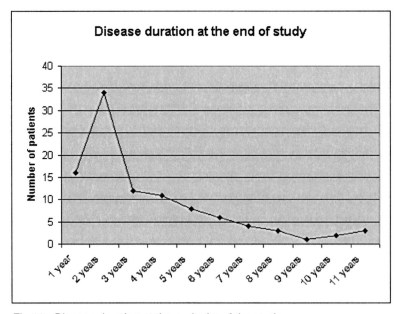

Fig.19 Disease duration at the endpoint of the study

In the great majority of patients (73%) the last examination was done in the first 4 years, while in the rest of 23 individuals in 5 up to 11 years after the reported disease onset. In none of these the worsening of disability, estimated according to Hoehn & Yahr staging, went concurrently with the duration of the disease. There was no statistical significant correlation between the duration of disease and the clinical stage on the Hoehn&Yahr scale (regression linear test $p < 0.05$). There was also no statistically significant difference, with regard to the disease duration, between patients with higher and those with lower Hoehn & Yahr clinical stage at the last neurological examination (one-way ANOVA $p < 0.05$).

Thus, in the followed up patients in the early stages of PD, and in the first years of its course, the disease duration did not influence the severity of Parkinson's disease.

Commonly, the severity of PD is clinically estimated on the basis of the Hoehn & Yahr staging. It is well known that the duration of the clinical stages Hoehn & Yahr, especially in the early stages, could be different from patient to patient. And also the severity of parkinsonian symptomatic in patients with the same clinical stage Hoehn & Yahr and with the same duration of disease could be different.

To estimate if the severity of PD is dependent from the intensity of the cardinal motor symptoms, and not only from the anatomical spread of these symptoms, there was considered of interest to investigate the correlations between the clinical stages Hoehn & Yahr and the UPDRS score of tremor, rigidity, bradykinesia, and postural instability.

Table 80

Follow-up more than 3 months

Correlations Hoehn & Yahr stages – UPDRS score

Number of patients

Changes of H & Y stage	Number of patients	Number of patients										
		Tremor			Rigidity			Bradykinesia			Post. instability		
		E=B	E>B	B>E	E=B	E>B	B>E	E=B	E>B	B>E	E=B	E>B	B>E
E = B	84	15	13	25	16	43	25	8	48	28	37	13	14
E > B	6	1	0	4	0	4	2	1	2	3	1	5	0
B > E	10	1	2	2	1	4	5	0	5	5	0	1	9

Legend

E = Last neurological examination

B = First neurological examination

The great majority of patients followed up more than 3 months was at the last neurological examination in the same Hoehn & Yahr clinical stage as at the first one (Table 80). There was a statistically significant correlation between the Hoehn &Yahr clinical stage and the the score of the motor cardinal symptoms (rigidity, bradykinesia, postural instability) but tremor at the last clinical examination (regression linear test p<0.05).

The tremor intensity did not influenced the Hoehn & Yahr clinical staging.
In the followed-up patients the Hoehn &Yahr stages correlated closest with the intensity and course of postural instability and rigidity, respectively.

In the early stages of PD the intensity of motor cardinal symptoms could fluctuate during the same Hoehn & Yahr clinical stage, as well as these stages could fluctuate in the same patient from one neurological examination to the next one.
Hence, the estimation of the disease severity should be better expressed by Hoehn & Yahr stage together with the UPDRS motor score and that of the disease progression must be done on the basis of a prolonged follow-up of at least 6 to 12 months.

Duration of early stages of Parkinson's disease

The attempt to estimate the duration of the early stages of the PD in untreated patients must take into consideration at least the following points:

1. The duration of the unilateral parkinsonian symptomatic,

2. The duration of the bilateral parkinsonian symptomatic without postural instability,

3. The duration of the bilateral parkinsonian symptomatic with postural instability.

There is generally accepted that the parkinsonian symptomatic usually begins unilaterally[134]. Some authors conditioned even the clinical diagnosis of the idiopathic Parkinson Syndrome (iPS) just from the unilateral onset of the parkinsonian symptomatic[253]. However, as Hoehn & Yahr[12] pointed out, a severe unilateral involvement is rare in patients with Parkinson's disease and more frequently in long-standing postencephalitic patients. As these authors noticed, the patients with Parkinson's disease usually develop bilateral signs before the disability is marked.

Of the 237 patients with untreated PS in this study 64, or 27%, reported anamnestically as the clinical onset of disease the appearance of an unilateral tremor. None of them reported an unilateral rigidity and/or unilateral bradykinesia as first signs of the illness. It seems that the rigidity and/or the bradykinesia when appearing unilateral as first symptoms of the disease commonly are not noticed by the patients. At the first neurological examination, 6 up to 24 months after the anamnestically noticed onset of the disease, 94% had already a bilateral symptomatic. Out of the 223 with bilateral symptoms 165 were without and 67 with postural instability in the pull test at the first neurological examination.

Some investigations with SPECT and DAT marker showed the presence of a bilateral striatum lesion even before this would be clinical manifest. So, Asenbaum S., Brücke T et al.[259], Seibyl JP et al[257], Marek KL et al.[258] found in patients with clinical hemiparkinsonism not only a diminished radioligands uptake in the DAT of the contralateral striatum but also a significant diminution in the DAT of the ipsilateral one, when no ipsilateral clinical parkinsonian symptomatic was yet present.

Therefore, there is to assume that the bilateralisation of the parkinsonian symptomatic is rather fast and in the majority of the patients it took place already before the patient consults a neurologist. As Hoehn & Yahr pointed out[12], the unilateral symptomatic could be skipped and no more found at the first neurological examination.

Of the 237 patients with untreated PD in this study the parkinsonian symptomatic was at the first neurological examination in 7 unilateral (Hoehn&Yahr stage 1), in other 7 unilateral & axial (Hoehn & Yahr stage 1.5), and in 223 bilateral corresponding to Hoehn & Yahr stage 2 (165 patients),or Hoehn & Yahr stage 2.5 (58 patients). The patients which presented at the last neurological examination still a hemiparkinsonian symptomatic had a disease duration from 6 to 48 months with a mean duration of 18.8 months and were observed up to 3 months after the first neurological examination. These data are in concordance with the observations of Hoehn & Yahr[12] which found in the majority of their cases with PD stage I (unilateral localisation) a duration of up to 4 years.

The patients in this study with unilateral & axial localization of the symptoms at the last neurological examination had a disease duration from 6 to 58 months. They could not be followed up longer because either they did not more come in the practice, or accepted an antiparkinsonian medication.

Out of the 100 patients followed up more than 3 months the great majority of patients with bilateral localisation (87%) remained in the same clinical stage during a disease duration of ½ year up to 11 years.

The data of this study showed that in the early stages of the Parkinson's disease, in the great majority of the patients, the generalization of the parkinsonian symptomatic is a rapid process which takes place in the first 1 to 2 years after the anamnestically reported clinical onset. Furthermore, taking into consideration the aforementioned data of the investigations with SPECT and DAT radioligands, it is to presume that the bilateralisation of this degenerative process is already present before the parkinsonian symptomatic became bilateral.

However, it remains unclear why in some cases (6% in this cohort of patients) the bilateralization of the parkinsonian symptomatic is slower and could be delayed months up to several years.

Thus, from the clinical point of view, the development of the Parkinson's disease seems to undergo firstly a phase of anatomical expansion of the parkinsonian symptomatic from unilateral, over an axial, to a bilateral involvement, followed by a phase marked by the appearance of a mild to moderate postural instability in pull test (Hoehn & Yahr stage 2). The appearance of an obvious postural instability with steady fall in pull test (when not caught by examiner), corresponding to Hoehn & Yahr stage 2.5, reflects a more severe stage of disease, which seems not to be dependent from the disease duration but rather from a more severe dysfunction of neural circuits involved in the maintaining of postural stability.

The mean disease duration of the followed-up patients at the endpoint of this study reached in those with Hoehn & Yahr stage 2.5 38.3 months with a statistical median of 25, and in stage 2 of the Hoehn & Yahr scale 37.13 months with a median of 23. There was no statistically significant difference in disease duration between patients without and those with obvious postural instability in pull test (one-way ANOVA p<0.05).

Taking into consideration the data brought by the observation of this cohort of patients, there is to assume that the early clinical stages of the Parkinson's disease are represented by the Hoehn & Yahr clinical stages 1, 1.5, 2 and 2.5 because in these stages takes place the anatomical spread of the clinical symptoms from unilateral to bilateral, the number of the cardinal motor symptoms can increase from at least two to four (bradykinesia, rigidity, tremor postural instability) in the stage 2.5, and the disease course is still fluctuating, i.e. from one neurological examination to the next, the intensity of the cardinal motor symptoms and even the presence of one of them (especially tremor or postural imbalance) is changeable.

Temporary changes from Hoehn & Yahr stage 2.5 to stage 2 and seldom from stage 2 to stage 1.5 could be still noticed in the early stages of PD. When such changes take no more place the severity of bradykinesia, rigidity, and especially of postural imbalance is progressive, the course of untreated Parkinson's disease reaches the "point of no return" namely the clinical stage 3 on the Hoehn & Yahr scale.

The course and duration of these stages could be variable from patient to patient. The causes are yet unknown.

Clinical criteria of therapy initiation

Although nowadays in the therapy of PD prevails the tendency the earlier the better, for the daily medical practice, there are yet no well established criteria for the right time to initiate a pharmacological therapy of Parkinson's disease. There are yet no biological markers for the Parkinson's disease which could faultless identify the presence of the illness either in the premotor or in the early clinical stages. Since the neuropathological studies of McGeer PL et al.[274] it is commonly accepted that the first clinical manifestations of the PD are appearing when 50–60% of the dopaminergic neurons in substantia nigra are lost. This process is presumed to last between 5 to 15 years, according to some, or 4 to 6 years according to other authors[7].

According to the neuropathological staging of PD proposed by Braak H et al.[275] the pathological onset of the Parkinson's disease would take place with the appearance of the Lewy bodies in the dorsal motor nucleus of the vagal and glossopharyngeal nerves or in the intermediate reticular zone and in the anterior olfactory nucleus or olfactory bulb. Accepting the point of view (still controversial) that the presence of Lewy bodies alone is the neuropathological hallmark of the Parkinson's disease, and supposing that they could appear before the loss of neurons in substantia nigra, the putting in evidence, in vivo, of the Lewy bodies in the central and/or autonomous nervous system would permit an earlier identification of the PD than PET or SPECT imaging of the DAT with radioligands. However such investigations do not yet exist.

Because also of that, in the past 2–3 decades the attention was focused to find out clinical signs and symptoms which could precede the appearance of the motor symptoms.

As such signs and symptoms are mentioned: olfactory disturbances, subtle neurocognitive dysfunction, visualmotor control, mood changes, personality disorders[6,7] or "idiopathic" REM sleep behavior disorders[276]. When a combination of some of them is present, that could lead to a PET or SPECT investigation with radionuclides.

However, on one hand, none of these premotor symptoms are specific for PD and, on the other hand, only in few patients with some of the aforementioned premotor symptoms, who were investigated with SPECT and radionuclides, were found a diminished binding of the radioligands to the DAT in striatum[277]. Therefore, in the majority of the patients the investigation with SPECT and radioligands either was done in a too early stage of the pathophysiological development of the PD, before the damage of the pars compacta of the substantia nigra, or the combination of premotor symptoms with SPECT + radionuclide investigation cannot evidence, in the great majority of the cases, the presence of Parkinson's disease.

Hence, the initiation of a pharmacologic therapy is exclusively a clinical decision and is depending on the presence and development on the cardinal motor symptoms.

Proceeding on the assumption that already in hemiparkinsonism a bilateral loss of dopamine transporter in striatum is present, as proved by studies with 123I-beta-CIT/ SPECT[258,259], the beginning of an antiparkinsonian therapy cannot be postponed, although there are yet not evidence based medicine studies which could prove that the early onset of pharmacological therapy could prevent or linger the bilateralization of the parkinsonian symptomatic in patients with unilateral symptoms. In the studied population of 237 untreated parkinsonian patients the very great majority (94%) had already at the first neurological examination a bilateral localisation of symptoms without or with postural instability. Less than 2% of them presented a temporary change of the bilateral localization to an unilateral & axial one.

On the basis of this study data, that is to consider the bilateral localization of the parkinsonian symptomatic usually as a not reversible stage in the development of the PD which makes necessary the initiation of an antiparkinsonian therapy independently from the UPDRS score.

Another criterion in the decision to begin a pharmacological therapy is the intensity course of the motor cardinal symptoms. The worsening of the symptoms severity would be reflected in the score of the subscales II and III of the UPDRS which are close correlated. In the majority of the patients followed up more than 3 months in this study the intensity of the motor symptoms and in few cases even the presence in the clinical picture of one or other of those symptoms varied during the observation. A worsening with 30% of the severity of one or more cardinal motor symptoms, according to UPDRS, between two successive neurological examinations in an interval of 3 to 6 months is a reason to initiate a pharmacological therapy.

Summarizing, the clinical estimation for the initiation of pharmacological therapy should take into consideration:

a. The localization of the symptoms,

b. The intensity of the parkinsonian symptomatic,

c. The progressive development,

d. The degree of disability in the activities of daily living.

However, these clinical criteria do not replace but lead to a L-Dopa test or a trial with a dopamine agonist substance for 2 to 3 months.

References

1.Martin WE, Loewenson RB, Resch JA, Baker AB, 1973,'Parkinson's disease, clinical analysis of 100 patients ' *Neurology,* vol.2, pp. 783-790.

2.Selby G, 1975, 'Parkinson's disease' *Handbook of Clinical Neurology* (ed.) Vinken PJ & Bruyn GW, vol. 6, pp.173-211.

3.Rajput AH, Stern W, Laverty WH, 1984, 'Chronic low-dose levodopa therapie in Parkinson's disease:an argument for delaying levodopa therapie' *Neurology,* vol.34, pp.991-996.

4.Hoehn M, 1992, 'The natural history of Parkinson's disease in the pre-levodopa and post-levodopa eras' *Neurologic Clinics,* vol.10(2), pp.331-339.

5.Koller WC, Langston JW, Hubble JP, Irwin I, Zack M, Golbe L, Forno L, Ellenberg J, Kurland L, Ruttenber AJ, 1991, 'Does a preclinical periode occur in Parkinson's disease?' *Neurology,* vol. 41(Suppl 2), pp.8-13.

6.Langston JW, Koller WC, 1991, 'The next frontier in Parkinson's disease' *Neurology,* vol.41(Suppl 2), pp.2-7.

7.Wolters EC, Francot C, Bergmans P, Winogrodzka A, Booij J, Berendse HW, Stoof JC , 2000, 'Preclinical (premotor) Parkinson's disease' *J Neurol,* vol.247 (Suppl 2), pp.103-109.

8.Berendse HW, Booij J, Stoffers D, Ponsen MM, Hijman R, Wolters EC, 2002, 'Presymptomatic detection of Parkinson's disease' *Tijdsch Gerontol Geriatr,* vol.33(2), pp.70-77.

9.Parkinson J, 1817, *'An essay on the shaking palsy'* London Sherwood, Neely and Jones .

10.Calne DB, Stoessl AJ, 1986, 'Early parkinsonism' *Clinical Neuropharmacology,* vol.9 (Suppl 2), S3-S8.

11.Bulpitt CJ, Shaw K, Clifton P, Sten G, Davies JB, Reid JL, 1985, ' The symptoms of patients treated for Parkinson's disease' *Clin Neuropharmacol,* vol.8(2), pp.175-183.

12.Hoehn MM, Yahr MD, 1967 'Parkinsonism: onset progression and mortality' *Neurology,*vol.17, pp. 427-442.

13.Jankovic J, 1992, 'Pathophysiology and clinical assessement of motor symptoms i Parkinson's disease' *Handbook of Parkinson's disease* 2nd Edn. Koller WC (ed) M.Dekker Inc. New York, pp. 129-157.

14. Jenkyn LR, Reeves AG, Warren T, Whiting RK, Clayton RJ, Moore WW, Rizzo A, Tuzun IM, Bonnet JC, Culpepper BW, 1985, 'Neurologic signs in senescence' *Arch Neurol*, vol.42(12), pp. 1154-1157.

15. Sandyk R, Fleming J, Brennan MJW , 1982, 'The head retraction reflex − its specifity in Parkinson's disease' *Clin Neurol Neurosurg*, vol.84, pp.157-160.

16. Bennet DA, Beckett LA, Murray AM, Shannon KM, Goetz CG, Pilgrim DM, Evans DA, 1996, 'Prevalence of parkinsonian signs and associated mortality in a community population of older people' *N Eng J Med*, vol.334(2), pp.71-76.

17. Fleischman DA, Wilson RS, Schneider JA, Bienias JL, Bennet DA , 2007, 'Parkinsonian signs and functional disability in old age' *Exp Aging Res*, vol.33(1), pp.59-76.

18. Louis ED, Luchsinger JA, 2006, 'History of vascular disease and mild parkinsonian signs in community-dwelling elderly individuals' *Arch Neurol*, vol.63(5), pp.717-722.

19. Barbosa MT, Caramelli P, Maia DP, Cunningham MC, Guerra HL, Lima-Costa MF, Cardoso F, 2006, 'Parkinsonism and Parkinson's disease in the elderly: a community-based survey in Brasil (the Bambui study)' *Mov Disord*,vol.21(6), pp.800-808.

20. Louis ED, Schupf N, Marder K, Tang MX , 2006, 'Functional correlates of mild parkinsonian signs in the community-dwelling elderly: poor balance and inability to ambulate independently' *Mov Disord*, vol.21(3), pp.411-416.

21. Louis ED, Tang MX, Schupf N, Mayeux R, 2005, 'Functional correlates and prevalence of mild parkinsonian signs in a community population of older people' *Arch Neurol*, vol.62(2), pp.297-302.

22. Murray AM, Bennett DA, Mendes de Leon CF, Beckett LA, Evans DA, 2004, 'A longitudinal study of parkinsonism and disability in a community population of older people' *J Gerontol A Biol Sci Med Sci*, vol. 59(8), pp.864-870.

23. Cosi V, Romani A, 1996, 'Neurologic findings in the normal elderly: prevalence and relationship with memory performance' *Aging* (Milano), vol.8(4), pp.243-249.

24. Weiner WJ,2005 'A differential diagnosis of Parkinsonism' *Rev Neurol Dis*,vol.2(3), pp.124-131.

25.Newman RP, Le Witt PA, Jaffe M, Calne DB, Larsen TA, 1985, 'Motor function in the normal aging population: treatment with levodopa' *Neurology,* vol.35(4), pp.571-573.

26.Calne DB, Peppard RF, 1987, 'Aging of the nigrostriatal pathway in humans' *Can J Neurol Sci,* vol.14(3 Suppl), pp.424-427.

27.Pearce JM , 1978, 'Aetiology and natural history of Parkinson's disease' *Brit Med J,* vol.2(6153), pp. 1664-1666.

28.Poewe WH, Wenning GK, 1996, 'The natural history of Parkinson's disease' *Neurology,* vol.47(6), pp.1465-1525.

29.Poewe WH, Wenning GK, 1998, 'The natural history of Parkinson's disease' *Ann Neurol,* vol.44(Suppl 1), pp.51-59.

30.Tetrud JW, Langston W, 1989, 'The effect of Deprenyl (Selegiline) on the natural history of Parkinson's disease' *Science,* vol.245(4197), pp.519-522.

31.Martilla RJ , 1992, ' Epidemiology' *Handbook of Parkinson's disease* 2nd Edn. Koller WC (ed) M.Dekker Inc. New York, pp.35-59.

32.Baba Y, Putzke JD, Wahley NR, Wszolek ZK, Uitti RJ , 2005, 'Gender and the Parkinson's disease phenotype' *Neurol,* vol.252(10), pp.1201-1205.

33.Angel RW, Alston W, Higgins JR, 1970, 'Control of movement in Parkinson's disease' *Brain,* vol.93, pp.1-14.

34.Joubert M, Barbeau A, 1969, 'Akinesia in Parkinson's disease' *Progress in Neuro-genetics* eds. Barbeau A, Brunette JR International Congress Series No.175 Amsterdam Excerpta Medica, pp. 366-376.

35,Hallet M, Khoshbin S, 1980, 'A physiological mechanism of bradykinesia' *Brain,* *vol.*103, pp.301-314.

36.Brumlik J, Boshes B, 1966, 'The mechanism of bradykinesia in parkinsonism' *Neurology,* vol.16, pp.337-344.

37.Marsden CD, 1984, 'The pathophysiology of movement disorders ' *Neurologic Clinics,* vol.2, pp.435-459.

38.Evarts EV, Terävainen H, Calne DB, 1981, 'Reaction time in Parkinson's disease' *Brain,*vol.104, pp.167-186.

39.Foerster O,1921, 'Zur Analyse und Pathophysiologie der striären Bewegungsstörungen' *Z ges Neurol Psychiat,* vol.73, pp.1-169.

40.Lee RG, Tatton WG, 1975, 'Motor responses to sudden limb displacements in primates with specific CNS lesions and in human patients with motor system disorders' *Can J Neurol Sci,* vol.2, pp.285-293.

41.Mortimer JA, Webster DD, 1979, 'Evidence for quantitative association between EMG strech reflexes responses and parkinsonian rigidity' *Brain Res*, vol.162, pp.169-173.

42.Rothwell JC, Obeso JA, Traub MM, Marsden CD, 1983, 'The behaviour of the long-latency strech reflex in patients with Parkinson's disease' *J Neurol Neurosurg Psychiat*, vol.46(1), pp.35-44.

43.Berardelli A, Sabra HF, Hallet M, 1983, 'Physiological mechanisms of rigidity in Parkinson's disease' *J Neurol Neurosurg Psychiatry*, vol.46(1), pp.45-53.

44.Bergui M, Paglia G, Lopiano L, Quattrocolo G, Bergamini L, Bergamasco B, 1995, 'Early modification of strech reflex in Parkinson's disease' *Acta Neurol Scand*, vol.88(1), pp.16-20.

45.Dick JP, Rothwell JC, Day BL, Wise RJ, Benecke R, Marsden CD, 1987, 'Modulation of long-latency reflex to strech by the supplementary motor area' *Neurosci Lett*, vol.75(3), pp.349-354.

46.Palmer E, Ashby P, 1992 'Evidence that long-latency strech reflex in human is transcortical' *J Physiol*, vol.449, pp.429-440.

47,Delawaide PJ, Sabbatino M, Delawaide C, 1986, 'Some pathophysiological of the parkinsonian rigidity' *J Neural Transm Suppl*, vol.22, pp.129-139.

48.Delawaide PJ, Pepin JL, de Noordhout AM, 1990, 'Parkinsonian rigidity: clinical and pathological aspects' *Rev Neurol*(Paris), vol.146(10), pp.548-554.

49.Cantello R, Gianelli M, Civardi C, Mutani R, 1996, 'Pathophysiology of Parkinson's disease rigidity.Role of corticospinal motor projections' *Adv Neurol*, vol.69, pp.129-133.

50.Delawaide PJ, Pepin JL, De Pasqua V, de Noordhout AM, 2000, 'Projections from basal ganglia to tegmentum: a subcortical route for explaining the pathophysiology of Parkinson's disease signs?' *J Neurol*, vol.247(Suppl 2), pp.75-81.

51.Tervainen H, Calne DB, 1980, 'Action tremor in Parkinson's disease' *J Neurol Neurosurg Psychiat*, vol.43, pp.257-263.

52.Koller WC, Vetere-Overfield B, Barter R, 1989, 'Tremor in Parkinson's disease' *Clin Neurophamacol*, vol.12, pp.293-297.

53. Kraus PH, Lemke MR, Reichmann HJ, 2007, 'Kinetic tremor in Parkinson's disease – an underrated symptom' *J Neural Transm*, vol.113(7), pp.845-853.

54. Uitti JR, 1998, 'Tremor: how to determine if the patient has Parkinson's disease' *Geriatrics*, vol.53(5), pp.30-36.

55. Elble RJ, 2000, 'Diagnosis criteria for essential tremor and differential diagnosis' *Neurology, vol.*54(Suppl 4), S2-6.

56. Rajput A, Robinson CA, Rajput AH, 2004, 'Essential tremor course and disability: A clinicopathologic study of 20 cases ' *Neurology*, vol.62, pp. 932-936.

57. Mc Auley JH, Marsden CD, 2000, 'Physiological, pathological tremors and rhythmic central motor control' *Brain,* vol.123(8), pp.1545-1567.

58. Djaldetti R, Mosberg-Galili R, Sroka H, Merims D, Melamed E, 1999, 'Camptocormia (bent spine) in patients with Parkinson's disease characterisation and possible pathogenesis of an unusual phenomenon' *Mov Disord* , vol.14(3), pp.443-447.

59. Lepoutre AC, Devos D, Blanchard-Dauphin A, Pardessus V, Maurage CA, Ferriby D, Hurtevent JF, Cotton A, Destee A, Defebre L, 2006, 'A specific clinical pattern of captocormia in Parkinson's disease' *J Neurol Neurosurg Psychiatry*, vol.77(11), pp.1229-1234.

60. Bloch F, Houeto JL, Tezenas du Montcel S, Bonneville F, Etchepare F, Welter ML, Rivaud-Pechoux S, Hahn-Barma V, Maisonobe T, Behar C, Lazennec JY, Kurys E, Arnulf I, Bonnet AM, Agid Y, 2006, 'Parkinson's disease with camptocormia' *J Neurol Neurosurg Psychiat*, vol.77(11), pp.1223-1228.

61. Slawek J, Derejko M, 2001, 'Camptocormia, a rare form of motor system disorders in Parkinson's disease' *Neurol Neurochir Pol*, vol.35(6), pp.1133-1340.

62. Azher SN, Jankovic J, 2005, 'Camptocormia: pathgenesis, classification, and response to therapie' *Neurology*, vol.65(3), pp.355-359.

63. Melamed E, Djaldetti R, 2006, 'Camptocormia in Parkinson's disease' *J Neurol*, vol.253(Suppl 7), pp.14-16.

64. Bonneville F, Bloch F, Kurys E, du Montcel ST, Welter ML, Bonnet AM, Agid Y, Dormont D, Houeto JL, 2008, 'Camptocormia and Parkinson's disease: MR imaging' *Eur Radiol*, vol.18(8), pp.1710-1719.

65. Duvoisin RC, Marsden CD, 1975, 'Note on the scoliosis of parkinsonism' *J Neurol Neurosurg Psychiatry*, vol.38, pp.787-793.

66. Jacobs JV, Dimitrova DM, Nutt JG, Horak FB, 2005, 'Can stooped posture explain multidirectional postural instability in patients with Parkinson's disease?' *Exp Brain Res*, vol.166(1), pp.78-88.

67. Bloem BR, Beckley DJ, van Dijk JG, 1999, 'Are automatic postural responses in patients with Parkinson's disease abnormal due to their stooped posture?' *Exp Brain Res*, vol.124(4), pp.481-488.

68. Goetz CG, 1986, 'Charcot on Parkinson's disease' *Mov Disord*, vol.1, pp.27-32.

69. Elmer L, 2005, 'Paralysis agitans- refining the diagnosis and treatment' *Parkinson's disease* Ebad M and Pfeiffer RF (eds.) CRC Press New York, pp.11-19.

70. Litvan I, Bhatia KP, Burn DJ, Goetz CG, Lang AE, Mc Keith I, Sethi KD, Shults C, Wenning GK, 2003, 'SIC task force of clinical diagnostic criteria for parkinsonian disorders' *Mov Disord*, vol.18, pp.467-486.

71. Jankovic J, 1991, 'Clinical aspects of Parkinson's disease' *Marsden CD New trends in the treatment of Parkinson's disease*, pp.53-75.

72. Brock S, Wechsler IS, 1927, 'Loss of righting reflex in man. With special reference to paralysis agitans ' *Arch Neurol Psychiat*, vol.17, pp.12-17.

73. Chaco J, Wolf E, 1970, 'Impairment of postural reflexes in Parkinson's disease' *Europ Neurol*, vol.4, pp.332-336.

74. Traub MM, Rothwell JC, Marsden CD, 1980, 'Anticipatory postural reflexes in Parkinson's disease and other akinetic rigid syndromes and in cerebellar ataxia' *Brain*, vol.103, pp.393-412.

75. Bloem BR, Beckley DJ, Remler MP, Roos RAC, van Dijk JG, 1995, 'Postural reflexes in Parkinson's disease during "resist" and "yield" tasks' *J Neurol Sci*, vol.129, pp.109-119.

76. Bloem BR, van Dijk JG, Beckley DJ, Roos RAC, Remler MP, Bruyn GW, 1992 'Altered postural reflexes in Parkinson's disease: a reverse hypothesis' *Medical Hypotheses*, vol.39, pp.243-247.

77. Reichert WH, Doolittle J, McDowell FH, 1982, 'Vestibular dysfunction in Parkinson's disease' *Neurology*, vol.32, pp.1133-1138.

78. Lakke JP, 1985, 'Axial apraxia in Parkinson's disease' *J Neurol Sci*, vol.69, pp.37-46.

79. Lakke JP, van Weerden TW, Staal-Schreinemachers A, 1984, 'Axial apraxia, a distinct phenomenon' *Clin Neurol Neurosurg*, vol.86, pp.291-294.

80. Steiger MJ, Thompson PD, Marsden CD, 1996, 'Disordered axial movement in Parkinson's disease' *J Neurol Neurosurg Psychiatry*, vol.61, pp.645-648.

81. Chou KL, Hurtig HI, 2005, 'Classical motor features of Parkinson's disease' *Parkinson's disease* Ebadi M and Pfieffer RF (eds) CRC Press New York, pp.171-181.

82. Batrolic A, Pirtosek Z, Rozman Z, Ribaric S, 2005, 'Postural stability of Parkinson's disease patients is improved by decreasing rigidity' *Eur J Neurol*, vol.12, pp.156-159.

83. Nallegowda M, Singh U, Handa G; Khanna M, Wadhwa S, Yadav SL, Kumar G, Behari M, 2004, 'Role of sensory input and muscle strength in maintenance of balance, gait and posture in Parkinson's disease: a pilot study' *AM J Phys Med Rehabil*, pp.898-908.

84. Beckley GJ, Panzer VP, Remler P, Bog LB, Bloem BR, 1995, 'Clinical correlates of motor performance during paced postural tasks in Parkinson's disease' *J Neurol Sci*, vol.132, pp.133-138.

85. Nova IC, Perracini MR, Ferraz HB, 2004, 'Levodopa effect upon functional balance of Parkinson's disease patients' *Parkinsonism Relat Disord*, vol.10, pp.411-415.

86. Bronte-Stewart HM, Minn AI, Rodrigues K, Buckley EL, Nashner LM, 2002, 'Postural instability in idiopathic Parkinson's disease: the role of medication and unilateral pallidotomy' *Brain*, vol.125, pp.2100-2114.

87. Bakker M, Esselink RA, Munneke M, Limousin-Dowsey P, Speelman HD, Bloem BR, 2004, 'Effects of stereotactic neurosurgery on postural stability and gait in Parkinson's disease' *Mov Disord*, vol.19, pp.1092-1099.

88. Rogers MW, 1996, 'Disorders of posture, balance and gait in Parkinson's disease' Clin *Geriat Med*, vol.12, pp.825-845.

89. Kemoun G, Defebre L, 2001, 'Gait disorders In Parkinson disease. Clinical description, analysis of posture, initiation of stabilized gait' *Press Med*, vol.30, pp.452-459.

90. Bloem BR, 1992, 'Postural instability in Parkinson's disease' *Clin Neurol Neurosurg*, vol.94, (Suppl.) pp.41-45.

91. van der Burg JC, van Wegen EE, Rietberg MB, Kwakkel G; van Dieen JH, 2006, 'Postural control of the trunk during unstable sitting in Parkinson's disease' *Parkinsonism Relat Disord,* vol.12, pp.492-498.

92. Adkin AL, Bloem BR, Allum JH, 2005, 'Trunk sway measurements during stance and gait in Parkinson's disease' *Gait Posture*, vol.22, pp.240-249.

93. Horak FB, Dimitrova D, Nutt JG, 2005, 'Direction-specific postural instability in subjects with Parkinson's disease' *Exp Neurol*, vol.193, pp.504-521.

94. Jacobs JV, Horak FB, 2007, 'Cortical control of postural responses' *J Neurol Transm*, vol.114, pp.1339-1348.

95. Gray P, Hildebrand K , 2000, 'Fall risk factors in Parkinson's disease' *J Neurosci Nurs,* vol.32, pp.222-228.

96. Dibble LE, Lange M, 2006, 'Predicting falls in individuals with Parkinson's disease: a reconsideration of clinical balance mesures' *J Neurol Phys Ther*, vol.30, pp.60-67.

97. Grimbergen YA,Munneke M, Bloem BR, 2004, 'Falls in Parkinson's disease' *Curr Opin Neurol*, vol.17, pp.405-415.

98. Adkin AL, Frank JS, Jog MS, 2003, 'Fear of falling and postural control in Parkinson's disease' *Mov Disord*, vol.18, pp.496-502.

99. Robinson K, Dennison A, Roalf D, Noorigian J, Cianci H, Bunting-Perry L, Moberg P, Kleiner-Fisman G, Martine M, Duda J, Jaggi J, Stern M, 2005, 'Falling risks in Parkinson's disease' *Neuro Rehabilitation*, vol.20, pp.69-182.

100. Cano-de la Cuerda R, Marcias-Jimenez AI, Cuadrado-Perez ML, Miangolarra – Page JC, Morales-Cabezas M, 2004,'Posture and gait disorders and the incidence of falling in patients with Parkinson' *Rev Neurol*, vol.38, pp.1128-1132.

101. Critchley EM , 1981, 'Speech disorders of Parkinsonism: a review' *J Neurol Neurosurg Psychiatry*, vol.44, pp.751-758.

102. Holmes RJ, Oates JM, Phyland DJ, Hughes AJ, 2000, 'Voices characteristics in the progression of Parkinson's disease' *Int J Lang Commun Disord*, vol.35(3), pp.407-418.

103. Dogan MI, Koseoglu M, Can G, Sehitoglu MA, Gunai DI, 2008, 'Voice abnormalities and their relation with motor dysfunction in Parkinson's disease'*Acta Neurol Scand*, vol.117(1), pp.26-34.

104.Hunker CJ, Abbs JH, Barlow SM, 1982, 'The relationship between parkinsonian rigidity and hypokinesia in the orofacial system: a quantitative analysis' *Neurology*, vol.32, pp.755-761.

105.Cole KJ, Abbs JH, 1983, 'Intentional responses to kinesthetic stimuli in orofacial muscles: implications for the coordination of speech movements' *J Neurosci*, vol.3(12), pp.2660-2669.

106.Caligiuri MP, 1987, 'Labial kinematics during speech in patients with parkinsonian rigidity' *Brain*, vol.110(4), pp.1033-1044.

107.Hanson DG, Gerratt BR, Ward PH, 1984, 'Cinegraphic observations of laryngeal function in Parkinson's disease' *Laryngoscope*, vol.94(3), pp.348-353.

108.Connor NP, Abbs JH, Cole KJ, Gracco VL, 1989, 'Parkinsonism deficits in serial multiarticulate movements for speech' *Brain*, vol.112(4), pp.997-1009.

109.Leopold NA, Kagel MC, 1997, 'Laryngial deglution movement in Parkinson's disease' *Neurology*, vol.48(2), pp.76-376.

110.Gamboa J, Jimenez-Jimenez FJ, Nieto A, Montojo J, Orti-Pareja M, Molina JA, Garcia-Albea E, Cobeta I, 1997, 'Acoustic voice analysis in patients with Parkinson's disease treated with dopaminergic drugs' *J Voice*, vol.11(3), pp.314-320.

111:Baker KK, Ramig LO, Luschei ES, Smith ME , 1998, 'Thyroarytenoid muscle activity associated with hypophonia in Parkinson's disease and aging' *Neurology* vol.51(6), pp.1592-1598.

112.Jiang J, O'Mara T, Chen HJ, Stern JI, Vlagos D, Hanson D, 1999, 'Aerodynamic measurements of patients with Parkinson's disease' *J Voice*, vol.13(4), pp.583-591.

113.Stelzig Y, Hochhaus W, Gall V, Henneberg A, 1999, 'Laryngeal manifestations in patients with Parkinson's disease' *Laryngorhinootologie*, vol.78(10), pp.544-551.

114.Jiang J, Lin E, Sheynin B, Hanson DG, 1999, 'Voice target time in Parkinson's disease' *Otolaryngol Head Neck Surg*, vol.12(11), pp.87-91.

115.Zarzur AP, Duprat AC, Shinzato G, Eckley CA, 2007, 'Laryngeal electromyography in adults with Parkinson's disease and voice complaints' *Laryngoscope*, vol.117(5), pp.831-834.

116.Gracco VL, 1988, 'Timing factors in the coordination of speech movements' *J Neurosci,* vol.8(12), pp.4628-4639.

117. Gracco VL, Abbs JH, 1988, 'Central pattering of speech movements' *Exp Brain Res,* vol.71(3), pp.515-526.

118. Logemann JA, Fisher HB, Boshes B, Blonsky ER, 1978, 'Frequency and cooccurrence of vocal tract dysfunctions in the speech of a large sample of Parkinson patients' *Speech Hear Disord,* vol.43(1), pp.47-57.

119. Shill H, 2005, ' Respiratory dysfunction' *Parkinson's disease* Ebadi M and Pfeiffer RF (eds) CRC Press New York , pp.323-327.

120. Miller N, Allcock L, Jones D, Noble E, Hildreth AJ, Burn DJ, 2007, 'Prevalence and pattern of perceived intelligibility changes in Parkinson's disease' *J Neurol Neurosurg Psychiatry,* vol.78(9), pp.1188-1190.

121. Ho AK, Iansek R, Marigliani C, Bradshaw JL, Gates S, 1998, 'Speech intensity in a large sample of patients with Parkinson's disease' *Behav Neurol,* vol.11(3), pp.131-137.

122. Murphy K, Corfield DR, Guz A, Fink GR, Wise RJS, Harrison J, Adams L, 1997,'Cerebral areas associated with motor control of speech in humans' *J Appl Physiol,* vol.83(5), pp.14328-1447.

123. Pinto S, Thobois S, Costes N, Lebars D, Benabid AL, Brousolle E, Pollak P, Gentil M, 2004, 'Subthalamic nucleus stimulation and dysarthria in Parkinson's disease: a PET study' *Brain,* vol.127(3), pp.602-615.

124. Wise RJ, Greene J, Büchel C, Scott SK, 1999, 'Brain regions involved in articulation' *Lancet,* vol.353(9158), pp.1057-1061.

125. Miyamoto JJ, Honda M, Saito DN, Ono T, Ohayama K, Sadato N, 2006, 'The representation of human oral area in the somatosensory cortex: a functional MRI study' *Cerebral Cortex,* vol.16(5), pp.69-675.

126. Brown S, Ngan E, Liotti M , 2008, 'A larynx area in the human motor cortex' *Cerebral Cortex,* vol.18(4), pp. 837-845.

127. Liotti M, Ramig LO, Vogel D, New P, Cook CI, Ingham RJ, Fox PT, 2003, 'Hypophonia in Parkinson's disease: neural correlates of voice treatment revealed by PET ' *Neurology,* vol.60(3), pp.432-440.

128. Smith MC, Smith MK,Ellring H, 1996, 'Spontaneous and posed facial expression in Parkinson's disease' *J Int Neuropsychol Soc,* vol.2(5), pp.383-391.

129. Simons G, Pasqualini MC, Reddy V, Wood J, 2004, 'Emotional and nonemotional facial expression in people with Parkinson's disease' *J Int Neuropsychol Soc,* vol.10(4), pp.521-535.

130. Ozekmekci S, Benbir G, Ozdogan FY, Ertan S; Kiziltan ME, 2007, 'Hemihypomimia, a rare persistent sign in Parkinson's disease' *J Neurol,* vol.254(3), pp.347-359.

131. Harding AJ, Stimson E, Henderson JM, Halliday GM, 2002, 'Clinical correlates of selective pathology in the amygdala of patients with Parkinson's disease' *Brain,* vol.25(11), pp.2431-2445.

132. Pollock M, Hornabrook RW, 1966, 'The prevalence, natural history and dementia of Parkinson'disease' *Brain,* vol.89, pp.429-448.

133. Mayeux R, 1992, 'The mental state in Parkinson's disease' *Handbook of Parkinson's disease* Koller WC (ed) 2nd Edn. M.Dekker Inc. New York, pp.159-184.

134. Fahn S, 2003, 'Description of Parkinson's disease as a clinical syndrome' *Ann N Y Acad Sc,* vol.991, pp.1-14.

135. Celesia GG, Wanamaker WM, 1972, 'Psychiatric disturbances in Parkinson's disease' *Dis Nerv Syst,* vol.33, pp.77-583.

136. Marttila RJ, Rinne UK, 1976, 'Dementia in Parkinson's disease' *Acta Neurol Scand,* vol.54, pp.431-441.

137. Hardyk C, Petrinovich LE, 1963, 'The pattern of intellectual functioning in Parkinson patients' *J Consult Psychol,* vol.27, pp.548 cited by Levin BE et al. 1989

138. Talland GA, Schwab RS , 1964, 'Performance with multiple sets in Parkinson's disease ' *Neuropsychologia,* vol.2, pp.85-93.

139. Levin BE, Llabre MM, Weiner WJ, 1989, 'Cognitive impairments associated with early Parkinson's disease' *Neurology,* vol.39, pp.557-561.

140. Lees AJ, Smith E, 1983, 'Cognitive deficits in the early stages of Parkinson's disease' *Brain,* vol.106, pp.257-270.

141. Cooper JA, Sagar HJ, Jordan N, Harvey NS, Sullivan EV, 1991, 'Cognitive impairment in early untrated Parkinson's disease and its relationship to motor disability' *Brain,* vol.114, pp.2095-2122.

142. Tröster AI, Stalp LD, Paolo AM, Fields JA, Koller WC, 1995, 'Neuropsychological impairments in Parkinson's disease with and without depression' *Arch Neurol,* vol.52, pp.1164-1169.

143. Mortimer JA, Pirozzolo FI, Hansch C, Webster DD, 1982, 'Relationship of motor symptoms to intellectual deficits in Parkinson's disease ' *Neurology*, vol.32, pp.133-137.

144. Globus M, Mildworf B, Melamed E, 1985, 'Cerebral bloodflow and cognitive impairment in Parkinson's disease ' *Neurology*, vol.35, pp.1135-1139

145. Cummings J, 1988, 'Intellectual impairment in Parkinson's disease: clinical, pathologic, and biochemical correlates' *J Geriatr Psychiatry Neurol*, vol.1, pp.24-36.

146. Emre M, 2004, 'Dementia associated with Parkinson's disease' *Lancet Neurol*, vol.2(4), pp.24-36.

147. Emre M , 2004, ' Dementia in Parkinnson's disease ' *Curr Opin Neurol*, vol.4, pp.399-404.

148. Williams-Gray CH, Foltynie T, Lewis SJ, Barker RA, 2006, 'Cognitive deficits and psychosis in Parkinson's disease: a review of pathophysiology and therapeutic options' *CNS Drugs*, vol.20(6), pp.477-505.

149. Emre M, Aarsland D, Brown R, Burn DJ, Duyckaerts C, Mizuno Y, Broe AB, Cummings J, Dickson DW, Gauthier S, Goldman J, Goetz C, Korczin A, Lees A, Levy R, Litvan I, McKeith I, Olanow W, Poewe W, Quinn N, Sampaio C, Tolosa E, Dubois B, 2007, 'Clinical diagnostic criteria for dementia associated with Parkinson's disease ' *Mov Disord*, vol.22, pp.1689-1707.

150. Albert 1974 ; Albert 1978   cited by Rafal RD et al. *Brain*, 1984

151. Rafal RD, Posner MI, Walker IA, Friedrich FJ, 1984, ' Cognition and the basal ganglia' *Brain*, vol. 107, pp. 1083-1094.

152. Aarsland D, Litvan I, Salmon D, Galasko D, Wenzel-Larsen T, Larsen JP, 2003, 'Performance on the dementia rating scale in Parkinson's disease with dementia and dementia with Lewy bodies: comparison with progressive supranuclear palsy and Alzheimer's disease' *J Neurol Neurosurg Psychiatry*, vol. 74(9), pp.1215-1220.

153. Maidment I, Fox C, Boustani M , 2006, 'Cholinesterase inhibitors for Parkinson's disease' *Cochrane Database Sys Rev*, vol. 20(6), CD004747.

154. Hakim AM, Mathieson MB, 1979, 'Dementia in Parkinson's disease: A neuropathological study' *Neurology*, vol. 2, pp.1209-1214.

155. Starkstein SE, Merello M, 2007, 'The unified Parkinson's disease scale: validation study of the mentation, behaviour, and mood section' *Mov Disord*, vol.22(15), pp.2156-2161.

156. Folstein MF, Folstein SE, McHugh PR, 1975, ' „Mini-mental state". A practical method for grading the cognitive state of patients for the clinician' *J Psychiatr Res*, vol.12(3), pp.189-198.

157. Muslimovic D, Post D, Speelman JD, Schmand B, 2005, 'Cognitive profile of patients with newly diagnosed Parkinson's disease' *Neurology*, vol.65(8), pp.293-1245.

158. Crum RM, Anthony JC, Bassett SS, Folstein MF, JAMA, 'Population-based norms for the Mini-Mental State Examination by age and educational level' *JAMA*, vol. 269(18), pp.2386-2391.

159. Dufouil C, Clayton D, Brayne C, Chi LY, Dening TR, Paykel ES, O'Connor DW, Ahmed A, McGee MA, Huppert FA, 2000, 'Population norms for the MMSE in the very old: estimates based on longitudinal data. Mini-Mental State Examination' *Neurology*, vol.55(11), pp.1609-1613.

160. Ferreri F, Agbokou C, Gauthier S, 2000, 'Recognition and management of neuropsychiatric complications in Parkinson's disease' *CMAJ*, vol.175(12), pp.1503-1519.

161. Kremer J, Starkstein SE, 2000, 'Affective disorders in Parkinson's disease' *International Rev of Psychiatry*, vol.12, pp.290-296.

162. Gupta A, Bahtia S, 2000, 'Depression in Parkison's disease' *Clinical Gerontologist*, vol.22(29), pp.59-70.

163. Starkstein SE, Merello M, Jorge R, Brockman S, Petracca G, Robinson RG, 2008, 'A validation study of depressive syndromes in Parkinson's disease' *Mov Disord*, vol.23(4), pp.538-546.

164. Mc Donald WM, Richard IH, DeLong MR, 2003, 'Prevalence, etiology, and treatment of depression in Parkinson's disease' *Biol Psychiatry*, vol.54(3), pp.363-375.

165. Aasland D, Irsen JP, Lim NG, Janvin C, Karlsen K, Tandberg E, Cummings JL, 1999, 'Range of neuropsychiatric disturbances in patients with Parkinson's disease' *Neurol Neurosurg Psychiatry*, vol.67(4), pp.492-496.

166. Pluck GC, Brown RG, 2002, 'Apathy in Parkinson's disease' *J Neurol Neurosurg Psychiatry*, vol.73(6), pp.636-642.

167. Micieli G, Tosi P, Marcheselli S, Cavallini A, 2003, ' Autonomic dysfunction in Parkinson's disease' *Neurol Sci*, vol.24(Suppl 1), pp.32-34.

168. Edwards LL, Pfeiffer RF, Quigley EM, Hofman R, Balluff M , 1991, 'Gastrointestinal symptoms in Parkinson's disease' *Mov Disord*, vol.62(2), pp.151-156.

169. Edwards LL, Quigley EM, Pfiffer RF, 1992, 'Gastrointestinal dysfunction in Parkinson's disease: frequency and pathophysiology' *Neurology*, vol.42, pp.726-732.

170. Byrne KG, Pfeiffer RF, Quigley EM, 1994, 'Gastrointestinal dysfunction in Parkinson's disease. A report of clinical experience at a single center' *J Clin Gastroenterol*, vol.19(1), pp.11-16.

171. Quingley EM, 1996, 'Gastrointestinal dysfunction in Parkinson's disease' *Seminars in Neurology*, vol.16(3), pp.245-250.

172. Hardoff R, Sula M,Tamir A, Soil A, Front A, Badarna S, Honigman S, Giladi N, 2001, 'Gastric emptying time and gastric motility in patients with Parkinson's disease' *Mov Disord*, vol.16(6), pp.1041-1047.

173. Pfeiffer RF, 2003, 'Gastrointestinal dysfunction in Parkinson's disease' *Lancet Neurology*, vol.2, pp.107-116.

174. Pfeiffer RF, 2005, 'Gastrointestinal function in Parkinson's disease' *Parkinson's disease* Ebadi M and Pfeiffer RF (eds.) CRC Press New York, pp.259-273.

175. Goetze O, Nikodem AB,Wiezcorek J, Banasch M, Przuntek H, Mueller T, Schmidt WE, Woitalla D, 2006, ' Predictors of gastric emptying in Parkinson's disease' *Neurogastroenterol Motil*, vol. 18(5), pp.369-375.

176. Norman L, 2005, 'Dysphagia' Pfeiffer RF (ed) *Parkinson disease and nonmotor dysfunction,* pp.93-104.

177. Chou KL, Evatt M, Hinson V, Kompoliti H, 2007, 'Sialorrhea in Parkinson's disease: a review' *Mov Disord*, vol. 22(16), pp.2306-2013.

178. Gurevich T, Korczyn A, Giladi N, 2005, 'Gastric dysfunction In: Parkinson's disease and nonmotor dysfunction' *Series Current Clinical Neurology*, Humana Press pp.105-114.

179. Bassotti G, Maggio D, Battaglia E, Giulietti O, Spinozzi F, Reboldi G, Serra AM, Emanuelli G, Chiaroni G, 2000, ' Manometric investigation of anorectal function in early and late stage of Parkinson's disease' *J Neurol Neurosurg Psychiatry*, vol. 68(6), pp.768-770.

180.TolosaE, Compta Y, Gaig C, 2007, 'The premotor phase of Parkinson's disease' *Parkinsonism Relat Disord*, vol.13(Suppl 3), pp.211-220.

181.Poewe W, 2008, ' Non-motor symptoms in Parkinson's disease' *Eur J Neurol*, vol.15(Suppl 1), pp.14-20.

182.Wakabayashi K, Takahashi H, Takeda S, Ohama E, Ikuta F, 1988, 'Parkinson's disease: The presence of Lewy bodies in Auerbach's and Meissner's plexuses' *Acta Neuropathol*, vol.76(3), pp.217-221.

183.Wakabayashi K, Takahashi H, Takeda S, Ohama E, Ikuta F, 1989, 'Lewy bodies in the enteric nervous system in Parkinson's disease' *Arch Histol Cytol*, vol.52(Suppl), pp.191-194.

184.Wakabayashi K,Takahashi, 1997, 'Neuropathology of autonomic nervous system in Parkinson's disease' *Eur Neurol*, vol.38(Suppl 2), pp.2-7.

185.Wakabayashi K, 1989, ' Parkinson's disease: 'The distribution of Lewy bodies in the peripheral autonomic nervous system' (English abstract) *No To Shinkei*, vol.41(10), pp.765-971.

186.Hess ChW, Enderli JB, Frölich-Egli F, Ludin HP, 1987, 'Neurogene Blasenstörungen beim Morbus Parkinson' *Nervenarzt*, vol.58, pp.55-60.

187.Singer C, Weiner WJ, Sanchez-Ramos JR , 1992, 'Autonomic dysfunction in men with Parkinson's disease' *Eur Neurol*, vol.32(3), pp.134-140.

188.Lemack JE, Dewey RBJr, Roehrborn CG, Suilleabhain PE, Zimmen PE, 2000, 'Questionnaire-based assessement of bladder in patients with milde to moderate Parkinson's disease' *Urology*, vol. 56(2), pp.250-254.

189.Sakakibara R, Shinotoh H, Uchiyama T, Sakuma M, Kashiwado M, Yoshiyama M, Hattori T, 2001, 'Questionnaire-based assessement of pelvic organ dysfunction in Parkinson's disease' *Auton Neurosci*, vol.91(1-2), pp.76-85.

190.Winge K, Wedelin LM, Nielsen KK, Stimpel H, 2004, 'Effects of dopaminergic treatment on bladder function in Parkinson's disease' *Neurourol Urodyn*, vol.23(7), pp.689-696.

191.Winge K, Skau AM, Stimpel H, Nielsen KK, Werdelin L, 2006, 'Prevalence of bladder dysfunction in Parkinson's disease' *Neurourol Urodyn*, vol.25(2), pp.116-122.

192.Singer C, 2005, ' Urinary dysfunction in Parkinson's disease' *Parkinson's disease* Ebadi M and Pfeiffer RF (eds.) CRC Press New York, pp.275-286.

193. Micieli G, Martignoni E, Cavallini A, Sandrini G, Nappi G, 1987, 'Postprandial and orthostatic hypotension in Parkinson's disease' *Neurology*, vol.37(3), pp.386-393.

194. Turrka JT, Tolonen U, Myllylä VV, 1987, 'Cardiovascular reflexes in Parkinson's disease' *Eur Neurol*, vol.26(2), pp.104-112.

195. Picha SL, Rinne O, Rinne UK, Seppänen A, 1988, 'Autonomic dysfunction in recent onset and advanced Parkinson's disease' *Clin Neurol Neurosurg*, vol.90(3), pp.221-226.

196. Meco C, Pratesi L, Bonifati V, 1991, 'Cardiovascular reflexes and autonomic dysfunction in Parkinson's disease' *J Neurol*, vol.238(4), pp.195-199.

197. Awebuch GI, Sandyk R, 1992, 'Autonomic dysfunction in the early stages of Parkinson's disease' *Int J Neurosci*, vol.64(1),:pp.-14.

198. Thomaides T, Bleasdale-Barr K, Chaudhuri KR, Pavitt D, Marsden CD, Mathias CJ, 1993, 'Cardiovascular and hormonal responses to liquid food challenge in idiopathic Parkinson's disease, multiple system atrophy, and pure autonomic failure' *Neurology*, vol.43(5), pp.:900-904.

199. Chaudhuri KR, Ellis C, Love-Jones S, Thomaides T, Clift S, Mathias CJ, Parkes JD, 1997, 'Postprandial hypotension and parkinsonian state in Parkinson's disease' *Mov Disord*, vol.12(6), pp.877-884.

200. Senard JM, Rai S, Lapeyre-Mestre M, Brefel C, Rascol O, Rascol A, Montastruc JL, 1997, 'Prevalence of orthostatic hypotension in Parkinson's disease' *J Neurol Neurosurg Psychiatry*, vol.63(5), pp.584-589.

201. Goldstein DS, Holmes C, Li ST, Bruce S, Metman LV, Cannon RO 3rd, 2000, 'Cardiac sympathetic denervation in Parkinson's disease' *Ann Intern Med*, vol.133(5), pp.338-347.

202. Kallio M, Haapaniemi P, Turkka J, Suominen K, Tolonen U, Sotaniemi K, Heikkilä VP, Myllylä V, 2000, ' Heart rate variability in patients with untreated Parkinson's syndrome' *Eur J Neurol*, vol.7(6), pp.667-672.

203. Goldstein D, Holmes CS, Dendi R, Bruce SR, Li ST, 2002, 'Orthostatic hypotension from sympathetic denervation in Parkinson's disease' *Neurology*, vol.58(8), pp.1247-1255.

204. Oka H, Yoshioka M, Onouchi K, Morita M, Mochio S, Suzuki M, Hirai T, Ito Y, Inoue K , 2007, 'Characteristic of orthostatic hypotension in Parkinson's disease' *Brain*, vol.130(Pt 9), pp.2425-2432.

205.Barbic F, Perego F, Canesi M, Gianni M, Biagiotti S, Costantino G, Pezzoli G, Porta A, Malliani A, Furlan N, 2007, 'Early abnormalities of vascular and cardiac autonomic control in Parkinson's disease without orthostatic hypotension' *Hypertension*, vol.49(1), pp.120-126.

206.Goldstein DS, 2006, 'Cardiovascular aspects of Parkinson's disease' *J Neural Transm* (Suppl), vol.70, pp.339-342.

207.Goldstein DS, 2006, 'Orthostatic hypotension as an early finding in Parkinson's disease' *Clin Auton.Res*, vol.16(1), pp.46-54.

208.Goldstein Ds,Sharabi Y, Karp BI, Bentho O, Saleem A, Pacak K, Eisenhofer G, 2007, 'Cardiac sympathetic denervation preceding motor signs in Parkinson's disease' *Clin Auton Res* vol.17(2), pp.118-121.

209.Mastrocola C, Vanacore N, Giovani A, Locuratolo N, Vella C, Alessandri A, Baratta L, Tubani L, Meco G , 1999, 'Twenty-four-hour rate variability to assess autonomic function in Parkinson's disease' *Acta Neurol Scand* , vol.99(4), pp.245-247.

210.Haapaniemi TH, Pursiainen V, Korpelinen JT, Huikuri HV, Sotaniemi KA, Myllylä VV, 2001, 'Ambulatory ECG and analysis of heart rate variability in Parkinson's disease' *J Neurol Neurosurg Psychiatry*, vol.70(3), pp.305-310.

211.Pursiainen V, Haapaniemi TH, Korpelainen JT, Huikuri HV, Sotaniemi KA, Myllylä VV, 2002, 'Circadian heart rate variability in Parkinson's disease' *J Neurol*, vol.249(11), pp.1535-1540.

212.Devos D, Kroumova M, Bordet R, Vodougnon H, Guieu JD, Libersa C, Destee A, 2003, 'Heart rate variability and Parkinson's disease severity' *J Neural Transm*, vol.110(9), pp.997-1011.

213.Kallio M, Suominen K, Haapaniemi T, Sotaniemi K, Myllylä VV, Astafiev S, Tolonen U, 2004, 'Nocturnal cardiac autonomic regulation in Parkinson's disease' *Clin Auton Res* vol.14(2), pp.119-124.

214.Oka H, Yoshioka M, Morita M, Onouki K, Susuki M, Ito Y, Hirai T, Mochio S, Inoue K, 2007, 'Reduced cardiac 123I-MIBG uptake reflects cardiac sympathetic dysfunction in Lewy body disease' *Neurology*, vol.69(4), pp.1460-1465.

215.Post KK, Singer C, Papapetropoulos S, 2007, 'Cardiac denervation and dysautonomia in Parkinson's disease' *Parkinsonism Related Disord*, vol. 14(7), pp. 524-532.

216. Davis TL, 2005, 'Disorders of thermoregulation in Parkinson's disease' *Parkinson's disease* Ebadi M and Pfeiffer RF (eds.) CRC Press New York, pp.319-327.

217. Pierangeli G, Provini F, Maltoni P, Barletta G, Contin M, Lugaresi E, Montagna P, Cortelli P, 2001, ' Nocturnal body core temperature falls in Parkinson's disease but not in Multiple-System Atrophy' *Mov Disord*, vol.16(2), pp.226-232.

218. Turkka JT, Myllylä VV, 1987, ' Sweating dysfunction in Parkinson's disease' *Eur Neurol*, vol.26(1), pp.1-7.

219. Saito H, Kogure K, 1989, 'Thermal sudomotor deficits in Parkinson's disease' *Rinsho Shinkeigaku*, vol.29(6), pp.734-740.

220. Kihara M, Kihara Y, Tukamoto T, Nishimura Y, Watanabe H, Hanakago R, Takahashi A, 1993, 'Assessment of sudomotor dysfunction in early Parkinson's disease ' *Eur Neurol*, vol.33(5), pp.363-365.

221. Hirashima F, Yokota T, Miyatake T, Hayashi M, Tanabe H, 1993, 'Sudomotor dysfunction in Parkinson's disease' *Rinsho Shinkeigaku*, vol.33(7), pp.709-714.

222. ManoY, Nakamuro T, Takayanagi T, Mayer RF, 1994, 'Sweat function in Parkinson's disease' *J Neurol*, vol.241(10), pp.573-576.

223. Yoshioka M, Oka H, Morita M, Inoue K , 2003, 'Sudomotor dysfunction in Parkinson's disease' *Rinsho Shinkeigaku*, vol.43(7), pp.379-384.

224. Shestasky P, Valls-Sole J, Ehlers JA, Rieder CR, Gomes I, 2006, 'Hyperhydrosis in Parkinson's disease' *Mov Disord*, vol.21(10), pp.1774-1748.

225. Shill H , 2005, 'Respiratory dysfunction' *Parkinson's disease*, Ebadi M and Pfeiffer RF (eds.) CRC Press New York, pp. 323-327.

226. Mosewich RK, Rajput AH, Shuaib A, Rozdilsky B, Ang L, 1994, 'Pulmonary embolism: an under-recognised yet frequent cause of death in parkinsonism' *Mov Disord*, vol.9(3), pp.350-352.

227. Wermuth L, Stenager EN, Stenager E, Boldsen J, 1995, 'Mortality in patients with Parkinson's disease' *Acta Neurol Scand*, vol.92(1), pp.515-522

228. Nakashima K, Tabata M, Adachi Y, Kusumi M, Ohishoro H, 1997, 'Prognosis of Parkinson's disease in Japan. Tottori University Parkinson's disease epidemiology (TUPDE) Study Group' *Eur Neurol*, vol.38(Suppl 2), pp.60-63.

229. Morgante L, Salemi G, Meneghini F, Di Rosa AE, Epifanio A, GrigolettoF, Ragonese P, Patti F, Reggio A, Di Perri R, Savetteri G, 2000, 'Parkinson's disease survival: a population-based study' *Arch Neurol*, vol.57(4), pp.507-512.

230. Beyer MK, Herlofson K, Aarsland D, Larsen JP, 2000, 'Causes of death in a community-based study of Parkinson's disease' *Acta Neurol Scand*, vol.103(1), pp.7-11.

231. Fall PA, Saleh A, Fredrickson M, Olsson JE, Granerus AK, 'Survival time, mortality,and cause of death in elderly patients with Parkinson's disease: a 9-year follow up' *Mov Disord*, vol.18(11), pp.1312-1327.

232. Vincken WG, Gauthier SG, Dollfuss RE, Hanson RE, Darauay CM, Cosio MG, 1984, 'Involvement of upper-airway muscles in extrapyramidal disorders: A cause of airflow limitation' *N Engl J Med*, vol.311(7), pp.438-442.

233. Tzelepis GE, McCool FD, Friedman JH; Hoppin FG Jr , 1989, 'Respiratory muscle dysfunction in Parkinson's disease' *Am Rev Respir Dis*, vol.139(2), pp.266-271.

234. Bogaard JM, Hovestadt A, Meerwaldt J, van der Meche FG, Stigt J, 1989, 'Pulmonary function in Parkinson's disease' *J Neurol Neurosurg Psychiatry*, vol.52(3), pp.329-333.

235. Izquierdo-Alonso JL, Jimenez-Jimenez FJ, Cabrera-Valdivia F, Mansilla-Lesmes M, 1994, 'Airway dysfunction in patients with Parkinson's disease' *Lung*, vol.172(1),pp.47-55.

236. Sabate M, Gonzalez I, Ruperez F, Rodriguez M, 1996, 'Obstructive and restrictive pulmonary dysfunctions in Parkinson's disease' *J Neurol Sci*, vol.138(1-2), pp.114-119.

237. Cardoso SR, Pereira JS, 2002, 'Analysis of breathing function in Parkinson's disease' *Arq Neuropsiquiatr*, vol.60(1), pp.91-95.

238. Korten JJ, Meulstee J, 1980, 'Olfactory disturbances in parkinsonism' *Clin Neurol Neurosurg*, vol.82(2), pp.113-118.

239. Ward CD, Hess WA, Calne DB, 1983, 'Olfactory impairment in Parkinson's disease' *Neurology(Cleveland)*, vol.33, pp.943-946.

240. Doty RL, Deems DA, Stellar S, 1988, 'Olfactory dysfunction in parkinsonism: a general deficit unrelated to neurological signs, disease stage, or disease duration' *Neurology*, vol.38, pp.1237-1244.

241.Doty RL, Stern MB, Pfeiffer C, Gollomp SM, Hurtig HI, 1992, 'Bilateral olfactory dysfunction in early stages treated and untreated idiopathic Parkinson's disease' *J Neurol Neurosurg Psychiatry*, vol.55, pp.138-142.

242.Pearce RKB, Hawkes CH, Daniel SE, 1995, 'The anterior olfactory nucleus in Parkinson's disease' *Mov Disord*, vol.10(3), pp.283-287.

243.Wenning GH, Shephard B, Hawkes C, Petruckevitch A, Lees A, Quinn N, 1995, 'Olfactory function in atypical parkinsonian syndromes' *Ann Neurol Scand*, vol.91, pp.47-250.

244.Hawkes CH, Shephard BC, Daniel SE, 1997, 'Olfactory dysfunction in Parkinson's disease' *J Neurol Neurosurg Psychiatry*,vol.62(5), pp.436-446.

245.Mesholam RI, Moberg PJ, Mahr RH, Doty RL, 1998, 'Olfaction in neurodegenerative disease: a metaanalysis of olfactory functioning in Alzheimer's and Parkinson's diseases ' *Arch Neurol*, vol.55(1), pp.84-90.

246.Sommer U, Hummel T, Cormann K, Mueller A, Frasnelli J, Kropp J, Reichman H, 2004, 'Detection of presymptomatic Parkinson's disease; combining smell tests, transcranial sonography and SPECT' *Mov Disord*, vol.198(10), pp.1196-1202.

247.Berendes HW, Ponsen MM, 2006, 'Detection of preclinical Parkinson's disease along the olfactory tract' *J Neurol Transm*, vol.70(Suppl), pp.321-325.

248.Quagliato LB,Viana MA, Quagliato EM, Simis S, 2007, 'Olfactory dysfunction in Parkinson's disease ' *Arq Neuropsiquiatr*, vol.65(3A), pp.647-652.

249.Louis ED, Marder K, Tabert MH, Devanand DP, 2008, ' Mild Parkinsonian signs are associated with lower olfactory test scores in the community-dwelling elderly' *Mov Disord*,vol. 23(4), pp.524-530.

250.Huisman E, Uylings HB, Hoogland PV, 2004, 'A 100% increase of dopaminergic cells in the olfactory bulb may explain hyposmia in Parkinson's disease' *Mov Disord*, vol.19(6), pp.687-692.

251.de Rijk MC, Tzourio C, Breteler MMB, Dartigues JF, Amaducci L, Lopez-Pousa S, Manubens-Bertan JM, Alperovich A, Rocca WA, for the EUROPARKINSON Study Group, 1997, 'Prevalence of parkinsonism and Parkinson's disease in Europe: the EUROPARKINSON collaborative study' *J Neurol Neurosur Psychiatry*, vol.62(1), pp.10-15.

252.Hughes AJ, Daniel SE, Kliford L, Lees AJ, 1992, 'Accuracy of clinical diagnosis of idiopathic Parkinson's disease: a clinico-pathological study of 100 cases' *J Neurol Neurosurg Psychiatry*, vol.55, pp.181-184.

253.Gelb DJ, Oliver E; Gilman S, 1999, ' Diagnostic criteria for Parkinson's disease' *Arch Neurol*, vol.56, pp.33-39.

254.Brooks DJ, 1991, 'Detection of preclinical Parkinson's disease with PET' *Neurology*, vol.41(Suppl 2), pp.24-27.

255.Brücke T, Podreka I, Angelberger P, Wenger S, Topitz A, Küfferle B, Müller CH, Deecke L, 1991, 'Dopamine D2 receptor imaging with SPECT: studies in different neuropsychiatric disorders' *J Cereb Blood Flow Metab*, vol.11, pp.220-228.

256.Vingerhoets FJ, Snow BJ, Lees CS, Schulzer M, Mak E, Calne DB, 1994, 'Longitudinal fluorodopa positron emission tomographic studies of the evolution of idiopathic parkinsonism' *Ann Neurol*, vol.36(5), pp.759-764.

257.Seibyl JP, Marek KL, Quinlan D, Sheff K, Zoghbi S, Zea-Ponce Y, Baldwin RM, Fussell B, Smith EO, Charney DS, Hoffer PB Innis RB, 1995, 'Decreased Single-Photon Emission Computed Tomographic 123I-beta-CIT striatal uptake correlates with symptom severity in Parkinson's disease' *Ann Neurol*, vol.38, pp.598-598.

258.Marek KL, Seibyl JP, Zoghbi SS, Zea-Ponce Y, Baldwin RM, Fussell B, Charney DS, van Dyck C, Hoffer PB, Innis RB, 1996, '123I-beta-CIT/SPECT imaging demonstrate bilateral loss of dopamine transporters in hemi-Parkinson's disease' *Neurology*, vol.46, pp.231-237.

259.Asenbaum S Brücke T, Pirker W, Podreka I, Angelberger P, Wenger C, Wöber C, Müller C, Deecke L, 1997, 'Imaging of dopamine transporters with iodine-123-beta-CIT and SPECT in Parkinson's disease' *J Nucl Med*, vol.38(1), pp.1-6.

260.Benamer TS, Patterson J, Grosset DG, 2000, 'Accurate differentiation of Parkinsonism and Essential Tremor using visual assessement of 123I-FP-CIT SPECT imaging: The 123I-FP-CIT study group' *Mov Disord*, vol.15(3), pp.503-510.

261.Catafau AM, Tolosa E, 2004, 'Impact of Dopamine transporter SPECT using123I-Ioflupane on diagnosis and management of patients with clinically uncertain parkinsonian syndrome' *Mov Disord*, vol.19(10), pp.1175-1182.

262. Eerola J, Tienari PJ,, Kaakola S, Nikkinen P, Launes J, 2005, 'How useful is 123I-beta-CIT SPECT in clinical practice?' *J Neurol Neurosurg, Psychiatry*, vol.76, pp.1211-1216.

263. Kish SJ, Shannak K, Hornykiewicz O, 1988, 'Uneven pattern of dopamine loss in the striatum of patients with idiopathic Parkinson's disease. Pathophysiologic and clinical implication' *N Engl J Med*, vol.318(14), pp.876-880.

264. Niznik HB, Fogel EF, Fassos FF, Seman P, 1991, 'The dopamine transporter is absent in parkinsonian putamen and reduced in the caudate nucleus' *J Neurochem*, vol.56(1), pp.192-198.

265. Brücke T, Djamashidian S, Bencsits G Pirker W, Asenbaum S, Podreka I, 2000, 'SPECT and PET imaging of dopaminergic system in Parkinson's disease' *J Neurol*, vol.247(Suppl 4), pp.IV/2-IV/7.

266. Lorberboym M, Treves TA, Melamed M, Lampl Y, Hellman M, Djaletti R, 2006, '123I-FP/CIT imaging for distinguishing drug-induced-parkinsonism from Parkinson's disease' *Mov Disord*, vol.21(4), pp.10-514.

267. Tolosa E, Coelho M, Gallardo M , 2003, 'DAT imaging in drug-induced and psychogenic parkinsonism' *Mov Disord*, vol.18(Suppl 7), pp.S28-S33.

268. Vaamonde J, Ibanez R, Garcia AM, Poblete V, 2004, 'Estudio pre et postsinaptico de la via nirgrostriada en el diagnostico diferencial del parkinsonismo en 75 patientes' *Neurologia*, vol.19(6), pp.292-300.

269. Kemp PM, 2004, 'Imaging the dopaminergic system in suspected parkinsonism, drug induced disorders and Lewy body dementia' *Nucl Med Commun*, vol.26, pp.87-96.

270. Suchowersky O, Riech S, Perlmutter J, Zesiewicw T, Gronseth G, Weiner WJ, 2006, 'Practice parameter: Diagnosis and prognosis of new onset Parkinson disease (an evidence-based review). Report of the Quality Standards Subcommittee of the American Academy of Neurology' *Neurology*, vol.66, pp.968-975.

271. Ravina B, Eidelberg D, Ahlskog JE, Albin RL, Brooks DJ, Carbon M, Dhawan V, Feigin A, Fahn S, Guttman M, Gwinn-Hardy K, McFarland H, Innis R, Katz RG, Kieburtz K, Kish SJ, Lange N, Langston JW, Marek K, Morin L, Moy C, Murphy D, Oertel WH, Oliver G, Palesch Y, Powers W, Seibyl J, Sethi KD, Shults CW, Sheehy P, Stoessl AJ, Holloway R, 2005, 'The role of radiotracer imaging in Parkinson's disease' *Neurology*, vol.64(2), pp.208-215.

272. Gotham AM, Brown RG, Marsden CD, 1986, 'Depression in Parkinson's disease: a quantitative and qualitative analysis' *J Neurol Neurosurg Psychiatry*, vol.49, pp.381-389.

273. Shrag A, Jahanshahi M, Quinn NP, 2001, 'What contributes to depression in Parkinson's disease' *Psychol Med*, vol.31, pp.65-73.

274. McGeer PL, Itagaki S, Akiyama H, McGeer E, 1988, 'Rate of cell death in parkinsonism indicates active neuropathological process' *Ann Neurol*, vol.24, pp.574-576.

275. Braak H, Del Tredici K, Rüb U, de Vos RAI, Jansen Steur ENH, Braak E, 2003, 'Staging of brain pathology related to sporadic Parkinson's disease' *Neurobiol Aging*, vol.24,pp.197-211.

276. Stiasny-Kolster K, Doerr Y, Möller JC, Höffken H, Behr TM, Oertel WH, Mayer G, 2005, 'Combination of "idiopathic" REM sleep behaviour disorder and olfactory dysfunction as possible indicator for alpha-synucleinopathy demonstrated by dopamine transporter FP-CIT-SPECT' *Brain*, vol.128(1), pp.126-137

277. Berendse HW, Booij J, Francot CM, Bergmans PL, Hijman R, Stoof J Wolters Ech,2001,'Subclinical dopaminergic dysfunction in asymptomatic Parkinson disease patients' relatives with decreased sense of smell' *Ann Neurol*, vol.50, pp.34- 41.